FACE LIFTING
BY EXERCISE

FACE LIFTING
BY EXERCISE

by SENTA MARIA RUNGÉ

ALLEGRO PUBLISHING CO.   POST OFFICE BOX 39892   LOS ANGELES, CALIFORNIA 90039

FIRST EDITION   -   April 1961

SECOND EDITION   -   October 1961

THIRD EDITION   -   June 1970

FOURTH EDITION   -   December 1971

FIFTH EDITION   -   September 1972

SIXTH EDITION   -   April 1974

SEVENTH EDITION   -   March 1976

EIGHTH EDITION   -   April 1977

NINTH EDITION   -   November 1980

Library of Congress Catalog No. A 526321
ISBN 0-9601042-1-6

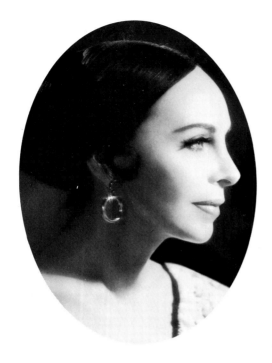

The Author

has devoted 23 years of research culminating in this book. Because of its underlying principle of muscle shortening, her method FACE LIFTING BY EXERCISE is the only one in the world by which one can lift a face naturally.

When Senta Maria Rungé, outstanding beauty authority, says, "You do not have to lose the beauty and youthfulness of your facial contour with the passage of years," she speaks with full confidence because she has proven her statement with countless women and men the world over.

She explains that what may appear as loose, flabby skin collecting at the laughline or in the lower cheeks, beside the chin, etc. are merely elongated upper cheek muscles that have lost their tone which is their elasticity or ability of holding up. The fine skin covering the flesh does not have the strength to hold up when the weight of the flesh moves and pulls downward. Although its elastic tissues have to surrender to the pull, the gratifying fact is that they will once more return to the size and shape of the muscle-flesh when that has been shortened through proper exercise.

As to how the system came into being, Senta Maria Rungé smiles and tells you, "It was born out of my own necessity." A European who endured privations during the years of World War II, it was those hardships of war that had begun to etch themselves on her face and neck when she was much too young for such aging. "I was only in my twenties when I suddenly realized that my neck was flabby and my face showed definite signs of sagging. I decided to try and find a way to stop the aging process if it was possible."

"Having been aware that the face is composed of muscles like the body whose firmness depends on adequate exercises - it was natural to me that only appropriate exercises could tighten up my relaxed facial muscles. Some people I knew were practicing grimaces and foolishly believed they were exercising their facial muscles. This I could never understand since reason and logic tell us that grimacing merely misforms muscles into lines, furrows and ugly features. Like myself I found others interested in this subject of learning more about the muscle structure of the face. Doctors, Dermatologists, Physical Therapists and Cosmeticians became challenged by the logical idea to exercise facial muscles in the search for the Fountain of Youth.

Madame Rungé says, "I myself undertook extensive research and study on this subject which included experiments on my face and constantly continue to do so." When she noted encouraging improvements, she confided her findings to a few close friends who followed her advice and were enthusiastic about the results. That was the beginning of a successful career which today helps countless women and men around the world.

The author says, "I have put my answers into a scientific formula of isometric exercises." She has surveyed the face into fourteen major muscle groups that, based on her knowledge contribute major contour defects upon relaxation. Of course, she says, "the structure is comprised of more muscles than I have included in my method, but those cause only minor problems and we would not find the time to exercise them all." From physical therapy she learned that one muscle movement in a long range of slow movements has many times the value than do many muscle movements in a short and consequently fast range. Her example is to lift your arms up once quickly (short range) and then once very, very slowly (long-slow-range movements) which will make you feel the difference. Based on this idea she was determined to find a way to resist all major muscle sections which would permit the longest and slowest muscle expansion possible.

Over a period of many years Senta Maria Rungé found an adequate resistance for all the muscle groups to her concern. According to her, those particular resistances permit us to impose the greatest effort on the muscles involved through the desirable long range movements. The blood circulation stimulated by the implied mechanical and chemical process brings about an instant shortening of the particular muscle sections which in turn means instant improvement to the exercised facial contour.

"I sometimes wonder why I am constantly challenged by this matter - however I do believe that we all are cut out for a specific goal and I am happy and proud to say that I have today the most advanced, comprehensive and effective method in facial contouring for retaining as well as for rehabilitating collapsed facial contours. To take all the credit for the accomplishments would be selfish and unfair. Doctors, Dermatologists, Physiological Institutes and others have contributed their building stones. My colleague, Helen Hede in Germany especially deserves great recognition for her knowledge and accomplishments in the area of facial exercises."

The author immigrated to the United States after World War II. There she made the American people contour conscious in 1959 when she introduced her method, FACE LIFTING BY EXERCISE, through a four-and-a-half page cover-line article in Vogue Magazine. That provocative story, which brought a new message and welcome encouragement to its readers, was followed up with a bestseller hardcover book, also titled FACE LIFTING BY EXERCISE in the Spring of 1961. Six months later the second edition had to be printed. In the Fall of the same year her popularity increased rapidly when, through a daily half-hour television program, she was able to demonstrate to the Southern Californians the effectiveness of her method. They had to be convinced, because — right before their eyes — they saw almost unbelievable transformations in the facial contours of her mature models, live on camera.

In the early sixties, Senta Maria Rungé opened the doors of her salon in Hollywood, through which walked the most famous personalities of the motion picture industry in search of their fountain of youth. The walls of her salon were covered with testimonials which she received from approximately 12,000 viewers who participated right in their own homes.

As an adjunct to her remarkable exercise technique, Senta Maria Rungé is also involved in research and the manufacture of unique and revolutionizing skin care products. These creations, she says, are as effective to the beauty of the skin as her exercises are effective to the beauty of the contour.

This busy woman has become a leader in the field of facial rejuvenation and has found time to raise a family of four.

HAROLD M. HOLDEN, M. D.
520 S. SAN VICENTE BLVD.
LOS ANGELES 48

Dear Madame Runge:

As a practicing plastic surgeon for over thirty years of experience, I have found that your work in facial exercises can play an important role in facial rehabilitation; and even more so in the avoidance of excessive wrinkling and sagging of the facial skin.

The surgical face-lift is the only procedure that can remove the excess sagging skin in advanced cases; but even after the most complete and extensive lift, it is not long before the vertical folds on the neck and under the chin reappear.

The facial exercises as advocated by you offer promise to prevent this recurrence after the surgical lift, and possible in many cases effect sufficient improvement that the lift could be postponed indefinitely.

Harold M. Holden, D.D.S., PH.D., M.D., F.I.C.S.
Los Angeles, Calif.

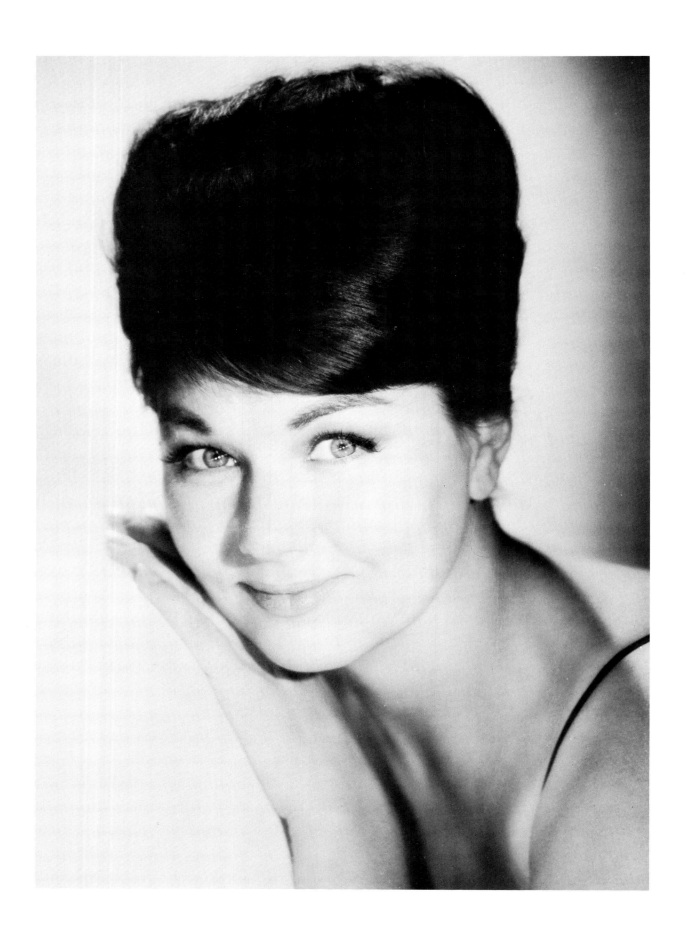

Beverly Hills, California

Dear Madame Runge:

About eight years ago I turned on the T.V. set and saw your program "Face Lifting By Exercise". The exercises didn't look hard and, as I had a couple of lines I didn't like, I tried them. I was so impressed and delighted with the immediately visible results that I have continued your exercises ever since.

As I am a professional entertainer even the tiniest facial lines are disturbing and could interfere with my career. I found that, in addition to the regular exercises, just before I went on stage, I could exercise out all of the visible small "tired lines".

I have a grown son who just completed a tour in the United Air Force. More than once while visiting him, we had the humorous problem of being accused of being newly weds.

I am very grateful for the help you have given me and for your kind friendship and advice on the use of your exercises and creams. I wish the same success to all who come in contact with you and your wonderful method.

Sincerely,

Laurie Loman Beinfeld

Laurie Loman Beinfeld

MY APPRECIATION

to John Engstead, for interpreting my method visually through his outstanding talent in photography,

to the models - who have been enthusiastic followers of my method for many years - for their ability and co-operation in demonstrating the exercises,

to my daughter Christine with great fondness for editing this book.

Thank you all!

CONTENTS:

Dear Reader 18
Man's Desire To Be Beautiful 20
CHAPTER I - Beauty And Aging Of The Face 23
Surgical Face Lifting 25
Other Beauty Surgeries Concerning
The Contour Of The Face And Neck 27
Skin Peeling 28
Injection Therapy 29
Other Beauty Surgeries Concerning The Face 29
Correction Of The Nose 30
Correction Of Receding Chin 30
CHAPTER II - Beauty Of Skin 31
Structure Of The Skin 31
Nature's Wonder 31
Beauty Of The Skin And Its Decline 32
What Causes Lines In The Skin 32
How Do We Distinguish Skin Creases From Contour Wrinkles 33
Factors Drying To The Skin 34
How To Retain A Beautiful Skin 36
How To Fight Against The Demons 36
Rainwater Compresses 37
CHAPTER III - Skin Care 39
A Program For Ultimate Skin Care 43
Cleansing Of Face And Neck 44
CHAPTER IV - Beauty Of Expression 51
The Power Of Expression 51
Your Expression Labels You 52
How To Express A Beautiful "YOU" 52

CHAPTER V — Beauty Of Contour 53
The Muscle Structure of Our Face 53
Youth Of Contour And Its Decline 54
Why Do We Have To Exercise Our
Facial Muscles Isometrically? 55
Can Isometric Exercises Be Substituted By A Machine? 56
What You Need To Know To Learn My Exercises 57
THE ULTIMATE OF EVERY EXERCISE IN MY METHOD 58
Necessary Skin Care When Applying My Exercises 61
Exercise Procedure 63
Tools Needed For Exercising 64
Exercise Rules 64
Can The Skin Be Stretched With These Exercises? 65
Working Example And Tips For Isometric Exercises 65
Facial Contours In Need Of A New Lease On Youth 68
How To Lift Your Face With A 10-Minute-A-Day Program 69
Expression Lines And Their Correction 71
Gaining Muscle Control 72
How Much Can One Expect From My Facial Exercises 74
How The Years Sneak Up On Us 77
Analysis Chart 78
Muscle Face 80

EXERCISES

Corrective Neck Exercises 82
Exercise No. 2 - JOWLS 98
Exercise No. 3 - BACK OF CHEEKS 104
Exercise No. 4 - LOWER CHEEKS 108
Exercise No. 5 - POUCHES 116
Exercise No. 6 - UPPER CHEEKS 122
Exercise No. 7 - UPPER LIP 134
Exercise No. 8 - LOWER LIP 140
Exercise No. 9 - FOREHEAD 144
Exercise No. 10 - SCOWL 148
Exercise No. 11 - UPPER EYELIDS 158
Exercise No. 12 - LOWER EYELIDS 164
                  - CROW'S FEET "IRON OUT" 170
Exercise No. 13 - CROW'S FEET 173
Exercise No. 14 - COMBINATION EYE EXERCISE 176
Exercise No. 15 - BRIDGE OF NOSE 180
Face-Ex 182
Excerpts from Testimonials 185

FACE LIFTING BY EXERCISE

by SENTA MARIA RUNGÉ

Dear Reader:

Could a 21 year old face possibly be lifted, to be given a more youthful contour? The answer is YES, of course the concept is a complete new revelation. Until recently, "Face lifting" was associated with the plastic surgeons knife only and thought to be exclusively for the "fallen face" that "suddenly" appears within the age of forty or fifty. The fact is that once the biological process of growing up is completed the face begins to change its contour en route "down". At the end of the teens the "baby fat" which cushioned the youthful soft roundness up to this time, gradually diminishes, thereby conveying the shaping of the face to the muscle structure beneath the skin, and so transforming the facial contour of a boy into a man's, and from a girl into a woman's.

Also imperceptible to the eye, this muscle structure changes constantly - perhaps daily - due to gradual elongation of the muscles responding to the gravity's pull. It is this gradual elongation of the muscle tissues that projects to the largest part the number of our calendar years. At 25 a face looks different than at 20, because the cheeks, the chin line and/or the eyelids have changed their position, they have slightly drooped down. The once high fitting "youth-full-ness" shifts downward leaving hollowness at the top and collecting (where it is not wanted) fullness at the bottom of the face (cheeks). The collapse of the upper cheek muscles alone may cause more than fifty percent of the aging appearance in the face. Consequently, elimination or correction of such collapse contributes equally to a younger look. Every tiny millimeter increase in the shifting downward of a muscle section, announces the sum total of birthdays.

18

Therefore, it is not the skin but the positioning of the muscle flesh beneath the skin which portrays a woman's or a man's age. Between the ages of 20 and 40, the upper cheek muscles may have elongated about one-half inch. By the age of 60, they may have elongated a full inch; the neck muscles about two inches, and the upper eyelid muscles about one-half to three-fourth of an inch.

Perhaps to us, by our tradition enslaved concept, the youthful contour at 23 could not possibly be promoted to more youthfulness, yet the cheeks if exercised as instructed in this book, will look firmer, higher up and also fresher. And I have seen such gratifying responses taking place in the most beautiful and youthful faces. The facial muscles, like muscles everywhere on our bodily structure need to be exercised to maintain their firmness and tone. My isometric exercises are designed to firm and to shorten elongated facial muscles, thus literally lifting a face regardless if 22 or 70 years old. The lifting possibility of course is determined by the degree of muscle elongation which depends largely on one's age. With each and every day that you apply one or more of my scientific facial exercises, you cannot help but see yourself looking younger since each correctly applied exercise in this book has the power to turn your clock back regardless of age. And if your contour can afford to eliminate 20 years from its appearance, this book can teach you how you may achieve this in three to four months.

Lack of beauty and its aging process is mere lack of knowledge. Therefore I hope that my happy message will reach everyone seeking to learn how to rejuvenate and to enhance the facial contour.

YOURS FOR BEAUTY

Senta Maria Rungé

Man's Desire To Be Beautiful

"The desire to look our best is an invitation to life and an expression of love and consideration toward our fellow men."

Man's desire to be beautiful and its supporting accoutrements are as old as mankind's history. According to archeological findings in caves reaching back to the Ice Age, lipsticks in the form of pointed, colored sticks were already in use by those inhabitants of approximately 70 million years ago. At that remote period and in what since has become part of the tradition of innumerable primitive tribes, the beautification processes in color and design were not limited to the face alone, but were extended also to the body. Such expressions for the desire to be beautiful were indulged in far more by men than by women. Camouflaging beauty tricks for the purpose of looking younger were already discovered and put to use by our ancestors long ago. Their aim, however, was not to attract the opposite sex but to deceive the enemy about the **warrior's age.**

The highest and oldest niveau of beauty culture so far as our modern concept is concerned was achieved by the Egyptians and dates back almost 5000 years. The great wealth of the Pharaohs made it possible for them to promote and indulge their love of beauty in that great cultural period. Since at the time it was believed that the King and Queen would return to this life, their burial places in the pyramids were piled high with evidences of great wealth and everything necessary for them to care for their beauty was lavishly provided. They did not, alas, return to use their treasures, but it was through those possessions that archeologists had opportunities of determining the extremely high cultural standard of the period. The scientific approach to skin and hair care, through creams and oils plus the realization of the importance of hormones, is approximately as old as that ancient Egyptian culture. Some of our ideas and practices in skin and hair care date back to that high cosmetic niveau when they were preserved on papyrus. Scientists and Cosmeticians are still making pilgrimages to the tombs, pyramids, museums, etc. hoping to find secret formulas among the hieroglyphs. Women in ancient times bathed in swan's fat, fresh wet leaves, rose water, rare spices and the very vain Empress Poppaea (Nero's second wife) bathed herself regularly in donkey's milk, presumably because she realized how friendly to the human skin milk is. It was, in fact, the Empress Poppaea who gave the first cosmetic advice and suggestions — written on papyrus and preserved until our time. Although beauty of face was at all times determined by the contour, skin and expression, so far as we know, it was only the skin that received attention and beauty care for its preservation. Even so the ideological concept for facial beauty has undergone periodic changes as to form and expression and consequently make-up, the beauty image of a woman's skin always has remained the same: cleanliness, tightness and tenderness. As long as women were sheltered from the world and did not have to go out and compete for a living, their most prized possession was a porcelain-doll appearance and they had sun-umbrellas, large hats, gowns extending down to the heels and up to the first vertebra, gloves protecting the hands from the sun's darkening rays, and bathing suits (when Milady ventured near the ocean) in knickerbocker length. Today's women may favor a fair complexion in winter, but during the summer months she prefers to sunbathe and let her body drink in healthful Vitamin D.

Nature very seldom creates a perfect masterpiece of a human being, usually it merely suggests or lays foundations for us to build and complete. Routines in achieving and presenting our good appearances have been built into our daily hygiene care for teeth, face, hair, nails, and other parts of the body. It is an indication of physical and mental health, a contribution to the happy environment of family, profession and social life. Therefore, regardless if woman or man, you owe it to yourself and to others to make and give the best of yourself. Looking our best does not project vanity as it was considered in former times, it expresses that we care for others and the refusal to so give expresses selfishness.

That the outer can change the inner, indeed the entire personality, has been proven to me over and over again in my salon in Hollywood. Drab, mousy, reticent girls, women and men who realized they had a facial imperfection but did not know how to correct it, have within a few weeks blossomed out and become almost a "new" person — alive, vital, happy, and optimistic. Being aware of imperfections gives one a very insecure feeling and that can be a great hindrance in life. It is my desire to give men and women everywhere a sense of self confidence about their facial appearance. For this I am grateful that with the information in this book I am able to help fill a void in the knowledge of the care of the face so that every man and woman can find assurance in their desire for facial beauty and this I am certain Y O U can do.

Although real beauty lies within — as a state of mind — it is the integration of the physiological and the psyche that makes up the image of the whole being. It has been said that a beautiful soul can exist only in a beautiful frame, which is the outer you, and that the soul can express nowhere more than in the face. We must realize, however, that to care for the outer body, to have it always look its best, we must be willing to work consistently in order to achieve what we hope for. Also the few who have been gifted by Nature with an exceptional abundance of beauty assets must work consistently to preserve those gifts. Through advanced medical and living standards, our span of life today averages twice what it was a century ago and out of this fact has been born the psycho-physical goal for adequately prolonged vitality and youth; hence beauty has become a science of international scope to biochemists, plastic and cosmetic surgeons, nutritionists, and cosmeticians. Whereas not too long ago the emphasis in the beauty industry was on skin enhancement, today's united scientific goal works toward preserving and regenerating tissues through tissue therapy and cellular life. The science of nutrition offers us longer life and youth due to the knowledge that the biological process of the human body is not toward inevitable disease but health which to a great extent is under our personal control. Modern science has estimated that compared with the life of animals the human span of life should average 100 years.

Chronological age is not and can not be a measurement of beauty, because beauty is ageless. A beautiful girl will maintain her beauty all her life providing she works for it. In fact, with the passing of years, she may actually mature in beauty and become even more lovely than in her younger years. Today when beauty aids are available to women and men in all walks of life, everyone who has the desire to explore the most attractive SELF also has the opportunity to attain this goal - through KNOWLEDGE.

And so, this book has been written to pass on to you the latest tools you will need to achieve your beauty goal, and equipped with this knowledge — you will be able to apply, explore and present the very best of yourself

FOR A MOST BEAUTIFUL AND HAPPY YOU!

CHAPTER I

Beauty And Aging Of The Face

Beauty and aging of the face depends on three factors: EXPRESSION — CONTOUR — SKIN. Each one of these subjects receives attention in this book.

BEAUTY OF EXPRESSION: Health, intelligence, calmness, kindness, "silent elegance".

AGING OF EXPRESSION: Tiredness, boredom, resignation.

REMEDY: Check your health and your diet. Find interest in life. Take an interest in an activity whereby you are helping your fellow man and in return you are appreciated and have a feeling of importance. It is a desire in all of us to feel needed.

As we enter a new season in life, new attractions, interests and fulfillments await us and new mental and spiritual support and strength is extended to us. Not wanting to realize or accept these gifts of life for each season and not making the best of them would be as foolish as not expressing the beauty of each season of life gratefully. If we understand the advancing years God grants us, then aging cannot mean fear but a new beauty for itself alone.

23

BEAUTY OF CONTOUR: Firmness and evenness.

AGING OF CONTOUR: Droopiness, flabbiness, wrinkles, furrows, hollowness, unevenness.

REMEDY: Isometric facial exercises as contained in this book.

BEAUTY OF THE SKIN: Cleanliness, smoothness, tightness, healthy texture, moisty and lustrous.

AGING OF THE SKIN: Dryness, cracks, lines, pale brownish color (terra cotta) listlessness due to lack of skin tone.

REMEDY: Cleanse, nourish and protect your skin with "proper" cosmetics. Tone and flabbiness can be improved best through isometric exercises that produce slow, long range expansion.

SURGICAL FACE LIFTING:

A general face lift includes the cheeks, jowls and mouth corners. (Some surgeons include also the neck.) The incision is made along the hairline on the forehead and the ears. The process consists of pulling the skin upward, tightening it and removing the excess skin. Surgical face lifting provides in most cases (at least temporarily) a good lift effect, however not in a natural form as one would wish. In order to be able to conceal the scars from the incision - by proper hair styling - the skin cannot be pulled and tightened according to its natural make-up, which is the way the skin is being moved by the underlying muscles. A very important consideration in this surgical skin cutting process is that too little rather than too much be taken away since too much may make the face appear "too" artificial and mask-like. A general face lift through skin cutting may look effective on your television or movie screen and in distance and may be preferred to a natural looking old wrinkled face. It must be understood however that surgery can never restore the tone to either the skin or the muscles. Therefore stretching the skin must be strictly avoided. The skin in the face may be compared to elastic fibers in a fabric. From the time the elastic fibers wear out, the fabric loses its shape. Perhaps the fit could be adjusted a few times by cutting down the excess, but, due to the lack of elasticity it will soon stretch again through wear. The duration of the lift effect in the face depends considerably on how much weight the skin has to carry. Consequently it stands to reason that a thin face receives more benefit from a lift than a fat face.

The tight skin obtained from a surgical face lift also gives the optical illusion of a contour lift, since it has been forced to hold up the underlying unelastic, lengthened, and droopy muscle flesh. But since the skin is not equipped for the job of holding the flesh ballast up, it soon conveys the responsibility back to the muscles where nature intended it to be.

More women and men consult plastic surgeons regarding face lifts because of droopy contour (muscle flesh) than for sagging unelastic skin. This is due to the fact that they do not understand enough about themselves. Most people do not realize what causes the condition that they desire to have corrected, nor do they have and get enough information as to the right method for the correction. What may appear as flabby loose skin on the upper and lower eyelids, on the furrows of laugh lines, on the pouches and bags beside the chin or on the neck, etc. are evidences of elongated facial muscles that have lost their tone, which is the elasticity of holding themselves firm and in shape. The skin is merely a thin covering over the flesh that has to go along with the muscle formation and alternately will return to the size of the muscle flesh when shortened through isometric exercises. The same symptoms of muscle elongation in form of flabbiness and droopiness also appear on our body wherever we have flesh. Who would ever consider plastic surgery to tighten skin for flabby upper arms, thighs or tummy? And yet it is exactly what women and men hope to have accomplished on the face. Flabby and droopy flesh is caused by muscles which have been ignored but fortunately muscles can always be tightened up again, through proper isometric exercises.

It should be understood that no plastic surgeon, and in fact nothing but exercises can tighten up unelastic muscles. Beneficial exercises cannot be administered by a machine or massage or any manipulations, only you by your own efforts can do it. The rule is: Surgical face lifting for unelastic skin by cutting away the surplus, and for unelastic muscle tissues isometric exercises which will shorten, thicken and restore the tone (elasticity) to the muscles and also a great deal to the skin. Assuming that the skin has not lost its entire elasticity - identified by its terra cotta color - the skin will then return with the muscles. In my practice, I have learned that many a woman who thought she needed her face rejuvenated through surgery only needed a change in her state of mind, based on the saying, "Lift the spirit and the spirit lifts the face." Most of the motives for such decisions are caused by an inferiority complex and frequently by the fear that the decline of what "used to be" could also cause the decline of those happy bubbles in the partner's champagne! Surgical face lifting performed on women who decide on this procedure with the hope of winning back the husband with whom a great part of the life has been shared, bear in most cases an unhappy end. With such partners the estrangement usually is of psychological nature and even the most favorable drastic change in a woman's face will therefore be meaningless. I personally have never known of an instance where a rejuvenation of a woman's face through beauty surgery brought reunification of a broken marriage. The greatest successes from surgical face lifting or other beauty surgery occur in those cases where the decision is brought about by the woman's desire to remove wrinkles and other signs from an aesthetic standpoint, especially if the face does not coincide with the heart. Another valid reason for undertaking such a procedure could be to start a completely new life because of certain circumstances. Such changes for the better may add a great deal of self-confidence so necessary in life's struggle and for that reason add to a better future.

OTHER BEAUTY SURGERIES CONCERNING THE CONTOUR OF THE FACE AND NECK:

N e c k : The removal of fatty deposits underneath the chin requires a surgery separate from the general face lift. In order to remove fatty deposits from this area the incision is made right beneath the chin. Skin tightening on the neck for the removal of turkey necks and flabby double chin(s) can look quite natural and beneficial. However, since the cause of the conditions is elongated unelastic neck muscles which cannot be remedied through surgery, the results from this procedure can only be enjoyed temporarily unless one shortens the muscles underneath the skin through proper isometric exercises. Once a woman whose career depended on public performances consulted me at the recommendation of her plastic surgeon after he had performed surgical skin tightening on her neck eight times!

U p p e r & L o w e r E y e l i d s : A general face lift does not include the lower or upper eyelids nor does it include the upper or lower lip and chin. Fatty deposits in the upper and/or lower eyelids causing puffiness or bags cannot be eliminated by exercises but only through plastic surgery. The removal of such fatty tissues and excess skin is considered a rather simple beauty surgery and if conscientiously performed, the results are very rewarding. After the fatty deposits have been removed, the surgeon pulls the skin on the lower eyelid upward and cuts away excess skin tissue. The incision is very close to the lower eyelashes and its fine scar is almost undetectable. The scar from the incision on the upper eyelids is usually so placed that it falls almost undetectable in a natural fold in this area. Puffiness in the upper and/or lower eyelids containing fluid (edema) cannot be removed surgically. For more information and understanding of this condition and its remedy refer to the eye exercise.

U p p e r & L o w e r L i p a n d C h i n : As mentioned in the "Exercise for Lower Lip and Chin", the muscular collapse in this particular structure expresses itself in the form of muscular atrophy (muscle disappearance). The entire upper lip, for instance, constitutes nothing other than a structure of muscle flesh covered by the skin. With the passing of time the muscle flesh becomes thinner, and thinner and we have seen pictures of people at an advanced age where the entire upper lip appears in the form of loosely hanging wrinkled skin. This process also applies to the lower lip and chin, but with the exception that the wrinkled crepe skin on the chin may rest on an underlying bony frame. The restoration of youth in those areas naturally does not call for skin cutting, hence the question is how to build up flesh. No surgeon can build up your muscle flesh, only you can do this through proper exercises. Since the decrease of muscle flesh causes the skin to shrivel and wrinkle, the plastic surgeon or dermatologist offers some help for this condition through skin peeling. Naturally this process affects only the appearance of the surface skin and in no way the shape of the lips or chin. The result from peeling off the wrinkled surface skin lasts only temporarily since the poor muscle condition beneath the skin very soon causes the same wrinkles to form into the new skin.

SKIN PEELING:

Whereas after a surgical face lift you still look at the same weather worn and marked skin - except a tighter one - the process of deep peeling a skin gives one a new and therefore clean and tight looking skin. The idea of the process comes from the desire to shed the skin like a snake letting the fresh new skin underneath take its place. For this reason a deep peel of the facial skin is sometimes preferred on those types of skin that displeased the bearer even before they started aging. The technique in this process involves the application of certain chemicals which work to separate and remove the outer layers of the skin. However, one should look into this treatment very carefully as it is considered unhealthy. The phenol used in this process goes through the skin into the bloodstream and may therefore cause harm, especially to the kidneys. Be certain that you choose only a qualified doctor if you decide to undergo this method of rejuvenation. It is pitiful how many unprofessional people do this kind of work and receive good fees for it. I have seen several cases where such attempts to peel off the facial skin have been made by laymen. In some, the faces were swollen for days, skin and muscles stretched, and even then the skin did not peel off satisfactorily causing the faces to fall into wrinkles altogether. On the other hand I have seen beautiful results from skin peeling. The new baby skin evident after the outer skin has been peeled off looks pink and somewhat artificial when compared to the rest of a mature appearance, but even so it gives a younger and more beautiful impression than does a dry, cracked skin. This we can have again later on. The new tight skin temporarily holds the contour of the face somewhat up, consequently giving it a rejuvenated look.

Unfortunately, the collapsed muscle structure beneath it soon pushes the new skin downward again which makes it necessary to repeat the "lift" unless one tightens and firms the facial muscles with proper isometric exercises.

My method of isometric facial exercises remedies the cause of the aging process of the face by tightening elongated muscles; thereby producing a lift where the contour has drooped, a firming up where the face appears flabby and a filling out by rebuilding atrophying muscle tissues. All this is done in a natural and healthy way, thus providing a natural youthful face which may be retained throughout life.

Many times I have been asked what the television and motion picture personalities do to keep young looking. Many of them (men and women) for the sake of their career had their face lifted surgically over and over, which can be quite natural and effective looking on the screen with proper theatrical make-up and proper lighting. However, it does not look so effective and natural in reality. Some performers hold their contour up during production by special tapes or clips which of course could not be worn on the street. Screen personalities that care for their youthful appearance outside their career have - like you and everyone else - no alternative but to consistently exercise isometrically their facial muscles in order to retain their youthful contour. Though I am not to mention their names, I wish to say that the stars (women and men alike) that really look young and beautiful for their age practice my method faithfully and treasure it as their secret.

INJECTION THERAPY:

It would be a wonderful therapy that could restore the youthful, even, firm form of the face simply by injecting a competent material to fill out where needed and to plump up the skin tissues! (All of this to be accomplished, of course, without any risk of health, pain of surgery, or work on our part!) Much experience and research has been and still is being conducted along this line in the hope of finding a satisfactory injection material. For some time now silicone has been used to "fill out". Some plastic surgeons object to having this foreign matter injected into our body tissues in the fear it may cause cancer or that the silicone will not stay put.

OTHER BEAUTY SURGERIES CONCERNING THE FACE:

The proper application of up-to-date beauty rituals in the privacy of our home make it possible for every girl and woman regardless of age, to present her face at its most attractiveness.

Medical science supplies us with beauty aids from within by correcting glandular and other disturbances and some beauty surgeons claim that there is really no visible anomaly of the face that could not be improved or corrected.

Each of the before mentioned beauty approaches contribute a substantial influence to our psycho-physiological status and self-confidence in our struggle for existence and this in turn reflects favorably on society in general.

The history of beauty surgery extends far back into antiquity at which time, so it is said, attempts were made in India to operatively correct facial anomalies, especially on the nose. Real progress along this line, however, was made possible through knowledge of asepsis. Today oriental eyes can be given occidental shapes by an operation requiring only a few minutes. Setting back protruding ears also is considered a minor operation. Perhaps the most common correction through surgery is rhinoplasty.

CORRECTION OF THE NOSE (RHINOPLASTY)

The correction of a nose through rhinoplasty is in all probability one that elicits the most gratitude of any form of beauty surgery, for it frequently changes the entire face and personality. A nose too long or too large has a tendency to give a more mature look, especially to a woman's face. Proper adjustments which bring about a harmonious relationship between nose and the rest of the face also implies a young appearance in most cases. The plastic surgeon is able to shorten long noses and slenderize wide ones, remove humps, and fill-up saddle noses. All these operations can be done from within the nose and, therefore, leave no visible scars. Not the least of the joys over the newly-formed nose is the assurance that the improvement is a lasting one. Many reputable plastic surgeons do not advise rhinoplasty before the age of 18, since through the growing period the facial form and personality change. Until the characteristics of a face are established, it is difficult to determine which shape of nose will best fit it.

CORRECTION OF RECEDING CHIN

Plastic surgeons counteract the distracting appearance of a receding chin by building it up through the insertion of a qualified material. The type of material used for this procedure changes with time, research, and experience. At the moment teflon is considered the most satisfactory material for this process, for along with many other considerations, whatever material used must be highly malleable for proper shaping.

CHAPTER II

Beauty Of Skin

STRUCTURE OF THE SKIN

The skin is composed of two basic layers:
a) a superficial layer called the epidermis
b) a deeper layer of connective tissues called the derma which is the true skin.

The epidermis is the very fine outer-skin layer which we can see and from where we are trying to remove the dead tissues with our daily cleansing procedure. New tissues are constantly and continuously being formed underneath and pushed upward where they die and have to be removed to make room for new tissues.

Embedded within the derma are the sebaceous glands (so important for our cosmetic purpose), the sweat glands, hair roots, nerve fibers and the tiny blood vessels, called capillaries. The sebaceous glands have the job of keeping our skin lubricated and soft. The tiny capillaries, which are shaped like hills curving up and down, have the function of delivering nutrients to every cell of the facial skin.

NATURE'S WONDER

Life comes from the sea, that great watery element from which, so the scientists tell us, all living things were formed. There is, according to these same scientists, the greatest kinship between our own blood and seawater, both containing the chemicals necessary to life and in their components being very similar. The native environment in the human's first form of life is water and out of the ONE-CELL-CAUSE have grown multimillion cells to form the human body. An average adult's skin alone has approximately ten million cells. To keep this highly complicated mechanism of Nature running smoothly is greatly in our own hands. Although we all come from ONE, and as ONE complex we are ONE, each varies from the other in all of its multimillion cells and so we distinguish individuals one from the other. To living matter, moisture is more important than food; for water is essential to carry on the life process. A man will perish of thirst long before he starves, a fact to which each individual cell contributes.

BEAUTY OF THE SKIN AND ITS DECLINE

Our baby skin, Natures birth gift was the most beautiful skin we ever possessed. Not everyone at birth is gifted equally by Nature. According to the law of inheritance, Nature favors some skins more than others depending largely on the moisture content in the skin. The tightness and plumpness of our skin is the result of the water content which accounts for approximately 75 percent of its make-up.

The skin is alive and renews itself constantly. The tempo of this process depends on the person's age. It is estimated that in a young person approximately eight million new cells are being processed daily. This production gradually declines with the passing years, bringing functional interruptions of the skin tissues and lack of activity of the oil glands, whereby the skin loses moisture and with it elasticity. We then have what we might term "Decline of Youth" in the skin. The aging process of a skin with its withering and flabbiness, cracks, lines and sagginess is mostly due to lack of moisture.

WHAT CAUSES LINES IN THE SKIN

Beauty of the skin and its lasting qualities depend on its moisture content. A child's skin does not etch lines from squinting, laughing or frowning, because a moist skin simply cannot crease as does a dry skin and the drier the skin the deeper the lines will etch. Extensive dryness may act so destructively on a skin that it actually causes cracks in the skin tissues. Clearly the aging process of the skin with its unattractive listlessness and lines is caused by lack of moisture. The drying process has not just started when it first becomes visible, as one might reasonably suppose; far more likely it started at the end of adolescence, with the exception of the oily skins. How many youngsters edge their crow's feet while skiing on snow or water or while otherwise playing out-of-doors? Such lines are a sign that valuable moisture in this skin area has escaped. Drying of the facial skin always starts on the sides (crow's feet area) and the very last part that wrinkles is the nose, since the oil glands at the center of the face are more abundant.

HOW DO WE DISTINGUISH SKIN CREASES FROM CONTOUR WRINKLES?

As mentioned previously, the beauty of the skin depends on its moisture content, and lines and creases in our skin are evidences of the lack of moisture. However, we must distinguish skin creases from contour wrinkles. Wherever in the face we are able to move the skin voluntarily, there are muscles attached to the inner layer of the skin. In everyone of these places where we move the muscles we have a potential line, fold, furrow or dimple. Those places are on the forehead where we have horizontal lines through lifting the eyebrows up and vertical lines between the eyebrows through pulling the brows together. Each line that appears is an indication of a muscular attachment, since without the muscles we could not move the skin and consequently could not get a line or wrinkle. Another area is underneath and on the sides of the eyes where squinting and laughing make lines. We are able to move our cheeks upward which causes the tiny muscles underneath the eyes to be pushed into wrinkles. By moving the laugh line (nose-mouth-line) upward we cause lines, since all four of the upper cheek muscles are attached to the skin in the laugh line. We can smile our lower cheek flesh backward just by the little curved vertical line beside each mouth corner which in a fatty and moist skin becomes visible only by smiling through pushing the mouth corners backward. However, once the baby fat in the mouth corner area diminishes, this little smile line will be visible at all times. Some people in their youth have dimples in the lower cheek when they smile - which in later years will show up as a line when the mouth corners are moved backward, which is an indication of a muscular attachment to the skin in the particular area. We see many wrinkles on the upper and lower lip when we purse, and each wrinkle or line appearing there gives us evidence that on this very spot there is a muscle attached to the skin. On the neck it is the horizontal lines that tell us the places of muscle location in the skin. When moving such a muscle and if the skin contains sufficient moisture, the muscular movements will not leave any trace; but when they do leave traces and tracks, one knows that the skin lacks moisture there. Those muscular movements leave creases in the skin. If the crease is deeper than on the mere surface skin, it is a contour wrinkle because the line is within the contour of the face. Since the contour of the face is determined by the muscle flesh underneath the skin and by the muscles partly attached to the skin, a contour wrinkle indicates a collapsed muscle or muscle group. All wrinkles can be corrected by proper exercises. In my practice I have known instances where women had beautiful moist skin in quite advanced years. Although the muscles underneath had collapsed and were shaky when moved, the skin had not creased, which evidenced its rich moisture content. But I regret to say that I have also seen young girls with perfect, youthful, firm contours but with creases in their skin put there from muscular movements, mostly from habit.

FACTORS DRYING TO THE SKIN

Sun and wind have drying effects on the skin. Perhaps this answers the frequently asked question from drivers as to why their left side of the face is drier and more wrinkled than the right side. Worst offenders in this drying process are the winds of spring and autumn and the seabreezes. A picture of an old Indian woman with her leathery-looking skin and the weather-beaten appearance of a seaman will show plainly what too much exposure to dry air or salty winds can do to the skin. Also, we know that people living in hot climates where the humidity is high, show age in their faces more quickly than those living in cooler climates and this is because the skin and muscles lose elasticity under the influence of the hot, damp air. In such climates the skin in a short time shrinks like silk under a hot iron. Hot steam bath which open the pores are good for deep cleansing purpose, but unless the skin is tightened afterwards with cold water will eventually shrivel up for the same reason.

As we know, sunlight is vital to life and summertime brings with it added health and beauty. But this is true only if moderation is practiced. Too much sun, especially if taken all at once may result in harmful damage to the skin. And, very confidentially, suntan is fashionable only until a certain age which the moisture content of a skin determines.

Dry, icy air, like moist heat, also is damaging to the skin. We have evidence of this from the Eskimos whose skins, even though protected with heavy grease, show the adverse effects of the climate in which they live.

Heat and ice, especially if applied directly to the skin, will tear down the tissues. Applying heat and ice to the skin may have temporary beauty effects, but in the end both are harmful.

It may surprise many readers to learn that water allowed to evaporate on the skin dries the skin. Proof of this are chapped lips and hands. Those living in cold climates may have at times experienced this fact to a degree that the skin of their hands bled from dryness inflicted by cold winds to which their insufficiently dried hands were exposed. I am certain, we all associate chapped lips with windy days. Due to the ever present moisture on the surface of our lips they not only look and feel dry, as does the rest of our facial skin, they actually chap when exposed to wind.

Allowing the salty ocean water after a swim to dry by air may be a temptation, but besides drying the skin, the sticky, salty sea water acts like glue to clog the pores. Also, the chemicals used to purify pools are particularly drying to the skin. Therefore, always rinse off with a fresh shower after swimming and dry the face and neck with a towel, since water allowed to evaporate on the skin dries the skin. Another successful and also widely practiced "drying treatment" on the facial skin is washing it with soap. Soap cleanses the skin by removing its surface oil, a process that obviously can be beneficial only for oily skins. Unfortunately - this method - although outdated since the discovery of cleansing cream - is commonly practiced on dry skins, which is like quenching fire with fuel. Shaving a dry skin with soap demands to be followed up with a moisturizing skin care product. A flaky and withered looking skin looks lifeless and unattractive in a woman's and a man's face alike.

Since the moisture content in one's skin determines its beauty and elasticity, it stands to reason that all measures be taken to preserve its moisture. At birth all skins are endowed with a reservoir of moisture that demands to be managed thriftily in order to enjoy its beautifying qualities for a long time. Therefore all precautions should be taken to prevent the moisture from escaping its deeper layers, since once it moves up to the surface it evaporates. Perspiration, regardless if triggered off through sunbathing, fever or facial steaming is drying to the skin because perspiration forces the skin's moisture to the surface. At the time, the moisture reaches the surface and until it has evaporated, it does lend the surface skin a youthful moist glow and one could easily be deceived by the impression that perspiration and steaming the facial skin are beneficial in moisturizing the skin. The fact is that the "true skin" beneath its superficial layers loses valuable moisture with each perspiration and therefore promotes its drying process.

Unfortunately, many "moisturizing" cosmetics and "temporary wrinkle removers" are based on the same deception. Their ingredients challenge the skin's moisture to the surface where it plumps up the tissues and minimizes at this point fine lines, and endows the skin with a moist youthful glow, until the moisture with its beautifying effects evaporates. All this is at the expense of the "true skin".

HOW TO RETAIN A BEAUTIFUL SKIN

The loss of beauty in the skin is due largely to the activity of the three demons:
1. Functional interruptions of the skin tissues, causing loss of moisture and consequently dryness and decreasing skin tone from within;

2. Negative climatic influences, causing dryness of the skin from without;

3. Negligent handling.

HOW TO FIGHT AGAINST THE DEMONS

DEMON NO. 1, the functional interruptions of the skin may be postponed by supporting bodily health through proper diet, since every cell in your body is built and nourished by the food you eat and the air you breathe. The skin's healthy look and lasting youthfulness depends on the support of the bloodstream which has to deliver the elements of health to the entire body. Activities, such as sports and exercises are important to stimulate and promote the delivery through the circulating blood. The vitality or decline of a facial skin depends much on adequate circulation produced by facial exercises. This process assures the maintenance of skin tone. Healthy blood is created by a wise selection of the food we eat. Since many books have been written on this subject, I will only briefly mention here the importance of vitamins for skin beauty. The vitamin B group is beneficial to the so-called "nervous skin" — a skin that is subjected to rashes caused by nerves. Vitamin B 1 (Thiamine) is helpful in preventing excessive oiliness. Vitamin A is recommended for dry skin and is sometimes called an inner skin lubricant; also it has been declared an eye beautifier. Additional aids to the skin are protein, calcium, lecithin and Vitamin E.

I must, however, advise our health conscious women and men that Vitamin E-oil belongs inside the body but not on the skin. Any oil applied to the facial skin is detrimental to the beauty of the skin. Not only does it give your skin a greasy look, it influences the oil glands adversely and relaxes the pores. Don't believe everything which sounds good — listen to your skin!

DEMON NO. 2 can be combatted with proper skin care. Cleanse, nourish and protect your skin as suggested under "SKIN CARE". Guard your skin against negative weather and climatic influences and avoid everything drying to the skin as outlined previously.

It is no secret that people living in cool, damp areas have the most beautiful skin - moist, tight and radiant. It may sound strange but even water has its own quality and some sources seem, for beauty purposes, to be better than others. Rainwater is the best, as even our gardens attest. In contrast to rainwater, our cultivated water contains a great amount of calcium and magnesium, both of which have drying effects on the skin. To prevent this drying action we have to soften our waters and this can be done by the addition of baking soda or boric acid. Even so, water thus treated does not have the same magical power for beautifying the skin that rainwater seems to possess.

RAINWATER COMPRESSES — NATURE'S MIRACULOUS COSMETIC FOR DRY SKIN

Since the results are cumulative one must apply those compresses daily for a period of two weeks. One gallon of rainwater as clean and fresh as possible (not cooked) is an adequate supply for one week of treatments. For the application the water should be at room temperature. Lie on a couch or slant board and beside you place a little stool at the level of your hands while you are lying down. On the stool place a large bowl containing one quart of rainwater in which you have soaked two linen or cotton towels to be used for the facial compresses, also one large terry wash cloth. The towels should be large enough to fold into two or three layers in order to retain more water. Protect your hair and the couch against the possibility of leakage. Within the reach of your hands have a bath towel folded many times and a face towel. One of the water soaked compress cloths covers the upper part of your face starting from the nose point to the hairline, the other covers the lower part of your face from ear to ear including the neck. Only the nostrils remain free for breathing. The compresses should be contoured by pressing tightly against the skin all over the treated area to avoid evaporation. Place the bath towel, folded several times, over the compresses to further keep the moisture from evaporating too fast. At approximately every seven to ten minutes add more rainwater to the compresses by squeezing the wash cloth gradually onto the compress at the middle of the face and cover up again with the bath towel. After every rainwater-compress cure, dry the facial skin thoroughly with a towel.

DEMON NO. 3 This demon can be fought with the slogan: "NEVER STRETCH THE SKIN". Regardless of skin quality, certain fundamental rules must be obeyed. For instance, careless stretching sounds the deathbell to lovely skin. Through the daily routines of washing, drying, creaming, applying and removing make-up, we handle our skin too much. Stretching the skin causes it, sooner or later, to sag. Supporting the "tired head" with the hand or sleeping on the face belong to the skin-stretching category. Another bad habit I have noticed is picking on the neck skin. The most sensitive skin on the face lies in the lower eyelid area and every little rubbing by hand or cloth will in a short time cause too much skin in this area. All manipulations on the skin must be made in such a way that the skin CANNOT be moved, because the skin can only be moved by stretching it. A child's skin when moved will always return to its original condition, because enough elasticity is present in the skin. But in order to prevent the child from developing a bad habit, it should be taught at an early age the proper way to wash and dry the skin without stretching it.

CHAPTER III

Skin Care

To maintain or to regain your youthful contour with my exercise method, without treating your skin for a youthful radiant texture, would be erroneous and from a beauty standpoint as incomplete as a face with a youthful looking skin covering a "fallen" contour.

The isometric exercises contained in this book have the power to remove contour wrinkles, firm up flabbiness, lift droopiness, support the elasticity of the derma (true skin), but they are not a substitute for proper skin care. The latter fact compelled me to engage in research, and in this pursuit I closed my studio in Hollywood in early 1970. Always challenged by the undiscovered and privileged with a unique gift, as you may surmise by reading this book, I became inspired with the desire to revolutionize skin care and to look for skin care aids, which, for the benefit of preserving the beauty and youthfulness of the skin, will allow us to maintain and to restore its normal process, which is the ultimate goal in skin care for any type of skin at any age, whether oily, dry or aged.

Since the cause of the skin's aging process is largely due to the loss of moisture as a result of the gradual disappearance of the skin's natural sealant, which constitutes its occlusive covering, the benefits obtained from moisturizers are accordingly limited in that they cannot prevent the skin from evaporating its valuable moisture. My quest therefore was to expand on the limited benefits moisturizers have to offer.

In 1977, I was able to announce a first breakthrough which I christened C-2 FOR NIGHT, the letter "C" representing a significant meaning which at this time I do not wish to divulge. The uniqueness of the C-2 lies in its ability to maintain as well as to restore the skin's natural sealant, a long quest in achieving the basic foundation for preventing its aging process.

C-2 FOR NIGHT is not a moisturizer in itself; it moisturizes through a unique process. First, it seals the skin, which may take several weeks. After the sealant has been established, C-2 slowly draws the natural moisture to the skin's surface, where it cannot escape and thereby allowing to regenerate tissues. As a result, a clear and youthfully radiant texture is achieved. C-2 FOR NIGHT also balances oily skins. However, it does not benefit the skin of the throat and lower eyelids due to the absence of oil glands in those areas. Since the C-2 is able to do its job only when the nervous system is in a relaxed state (during sleep), a corresponding product for the day had to be discovered.

In December 1978, I was then able to introduce the C-3 FOR DAY. Like its forerunner, the C-3 was another breakthrough in the cosmetic industry, distinguishing itself in its composition and performance from all other skin care products available anywhere. C-3 consists of two parts. Part I is a cream which uniquely nourishes and strengthens the skin. Its performance, however, depends on its activator, a lotion, which is Part II. This ally seals the cream into the skin for six hours, constantly activating the cream to do its work. The dual process not only helps to prevent the skin's aging process, but it also has the capacity to lend it a youthfully radiant texture by vitalizing, nourishing, moisturizing and building up skin. In addition it protects against climatic influences, tightens pores and strengthens tissues. Because of its unique balancing capability, the C-3 FOR DAY, like its predecessor, is beneficial to all types of skin for any age and serves oily as well as dry skin. The activating lotion may be worn under as well as over make-up. Men find the C-3 an unsurpassed after-shave product, since it nourishes and builds up the skin while at the same time it refreshens and tightens the pores. Astringents and after-shave lotions can tighten pores only for 10-20 minutes maximum, the C-3 Activator does the job for 6 hours. The C-3 FOR DAY usually presents its first testimonial after only 3 days by lending the skin a clearer, tighter and more radiant texture.

The holistic skin care concept I had been aiming for reached its achievement in 1979, when I introduced the C-5 NUTRI MASK. This product not only prepares the skin for the ultimate achievements of the C-2 and C-3, it is also a special skin food for all types of skin, whether dry, oily or normal. Because the C-5 supplies the missing link in mineral nourishment, it renews and facilitates the skin's normal process. C-5 cleanses from deep within and aids in removing impurities such as blackheads and whiteheads, while at the same time it balances oiliness. It is a known fact that conventional masks have a drying effect upon the skin. Hence dry skin should not be subjected to such applications. Unlike conventional masks, the C-5 NUTRI MASK is especially beneficial for aged, as well as acne troubled adolescent skin because it facilitates the revitalization of the skin's tissue and the balancing of the skin's chemistry. Skin abused by excessive sun exposure (not sunburn) may show an unbelievable transformation from just one application of the C-5 NUTRI MASK.

The benefits obtainable through the C-Products exceed by far those obtainable through moisturizers in that they uniquely prevent the aging process of the skin which is caused by the evaporation of its moisture. I am happy to say that as a result of my success with the holistic C-TRIO, these skin care aids are as effective to the beauty of the skin as my exercises are effective to the beauty of the contour. Only natural ingredients are used in the TRIO, except for the necessary preservatives, which must be added to protect the user from bacterial contamination and to increase the efficacy of the products.

My readers may wonder what happened with the C-1, C-4, and C-6. At the time this section of the book was prepared for the 9th edition, the missing links in the C-Chain were still in the "cauldron" awaiting perfection. The C-1, if completed, will take care of pigment disorders, such as brown spots, etc. C-4, if completed, will introduce a much desired, yet totally new concept in natural skin enhancement. From an aesthetic point of view, the C-6, if completed, will bring the greatest blessing to mankind.

You may request an order brochure by writing to the address below, but please do not ask us to inform you about completed products. You will be automatically advised through our circulars if you are an established patron of Rungé Cosmetics.

MME. RUNGÉ COSMETICS, INC.
P.O. Box 39523
Hollywood, California 90039

A PROGRAM FOR ULTIMATE SKIN CARE

M O R N I N G S :   Cleanse — Nourish — Protect.

CLEANSING: Cleanse skin with a water soluble Cleansing Cream to remove dead tissues which have pushed to the surface during the night. "Bumpy", tired and unclear looking skin usually testifies to the absence of this necessary process. The C-2, C-3 and C-5 will do the job of cleansing from within and the Cleansing Cream from without. If the Cleansing Cream is water soluble there is no need to follow up with an Astringent because it can be removed thoroughly with water. Astringents or any other application would interfere with the function of the C-Products.

NOURISHING: Apply C-3 CREAM FOR DAY over face and throat.

PROTECTING: Apply C-3 ACTIVATOR over creamed area. Reapply ACTIVATOR every six hours. The difference between one or two applications is as different as day and night.

E V E N I N G S :   Cleanse — Nourish.

CLEANSING: Cleanse skin thoroughly as above if make-up has been used.

NOURISHING: Apply C-2 FOR NIGHT, alternating with C-5 NUTRI MASK. Treat throat skin with our unique Tears of Venus Throat Oil in conjunction with a moisturizing cream. According to the findings of European bio-chemists, the throat skin needs to be treated with Oil **and** Moisture because it lacks oil glands in that particular area, a condition responsible for crepe skin. Treat lower eyelids, lashes and lips with Runge Cosmetics Eye-Lip-Dew.

Cleansing Of Face And Neck
As You Prepare For The Exercises

When cleansing and creaming your face and neck picture your skin as a structure of scales - like the skin of a fish. Therefore, in order to cleanse and to nourish the skin properly, one has to apply those treatments in UPWARD strokes thus reaching "under" the scales. When applying make-up and powder, the finish strokes must be downward to give the skin a smooth look.

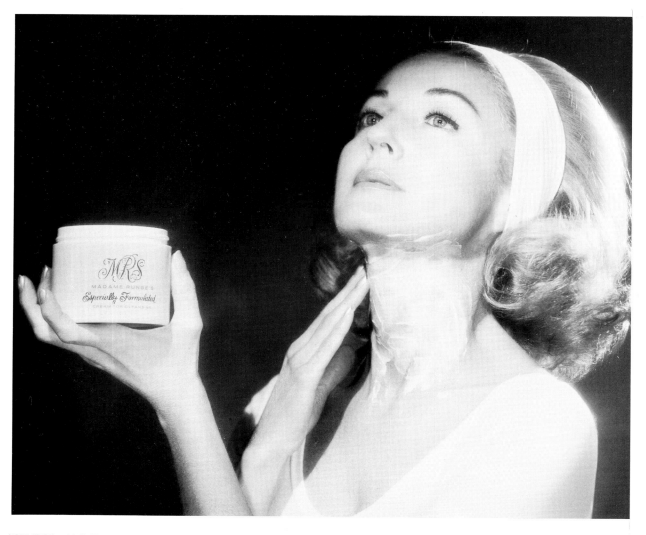

NECK: While cleansing, drying or creaming, hold your chin U P , so the neck muscles will keep the skin taut while you work on it. Your neck-skin must be completely immobile in this position.

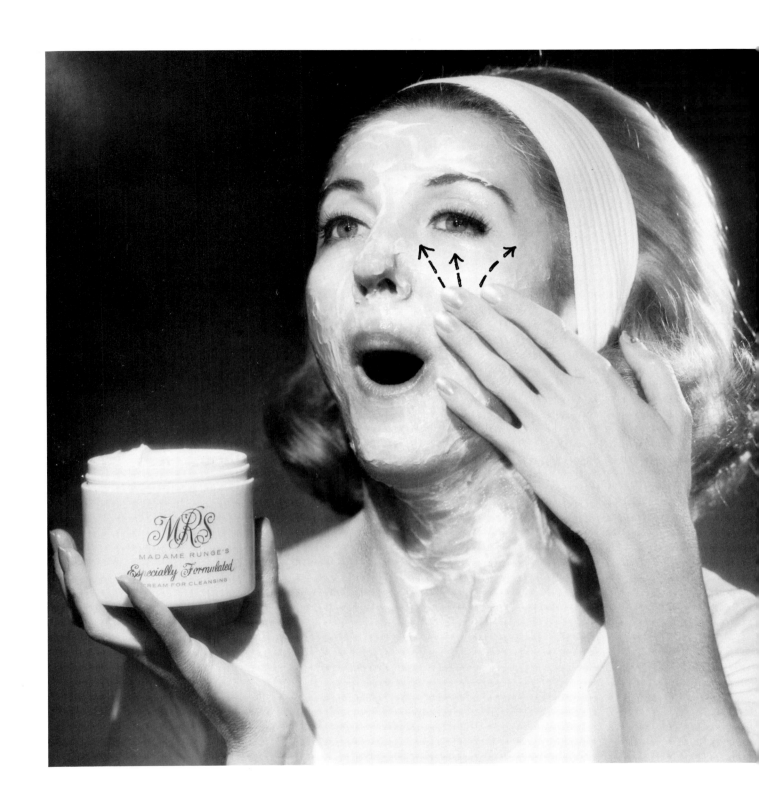

CHEEKS: When working on the cheeks, draw jaw and upper lip down. Do NOT permit an OVAL in your mouth position. The skin in this position must be immobile.

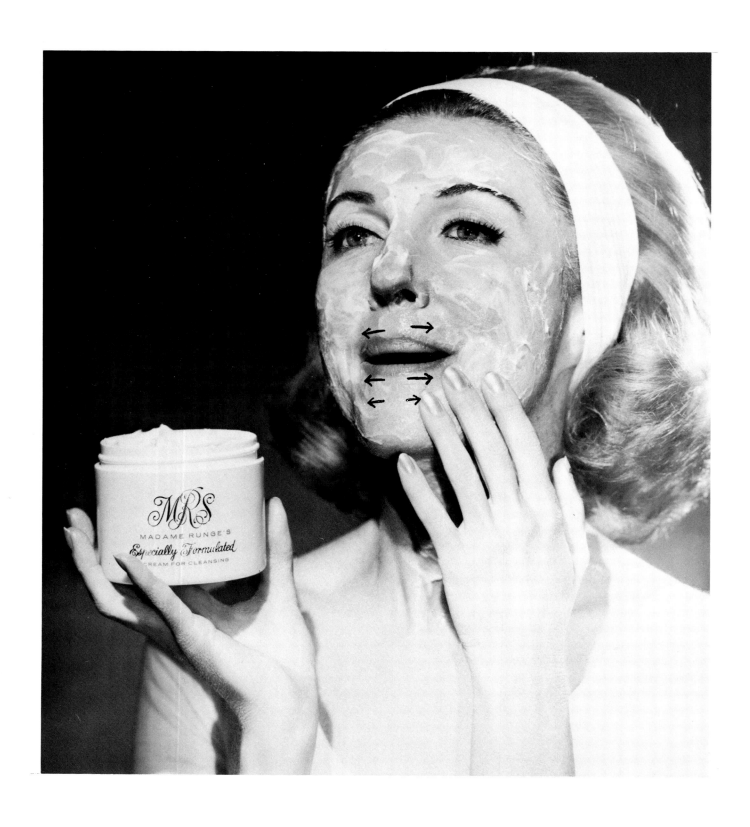

CHIN & LIPS: Tighten the skin by pulling chin and lip muscles apart, move upper lip slightly down.

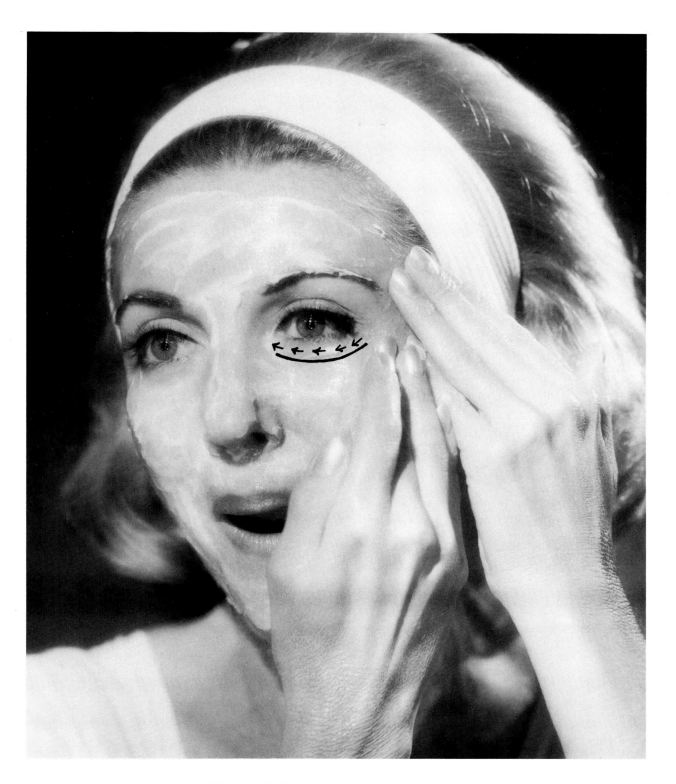

LOWER EYELIDS: When working on the lower eyelids hold them in a taut position by holding jaw and upper lip down without forming an oval. Squint slightly upward and hold your skin in the temple area against the bone. Work on the lower eyelids by moving with one or two fingers toward the nose.

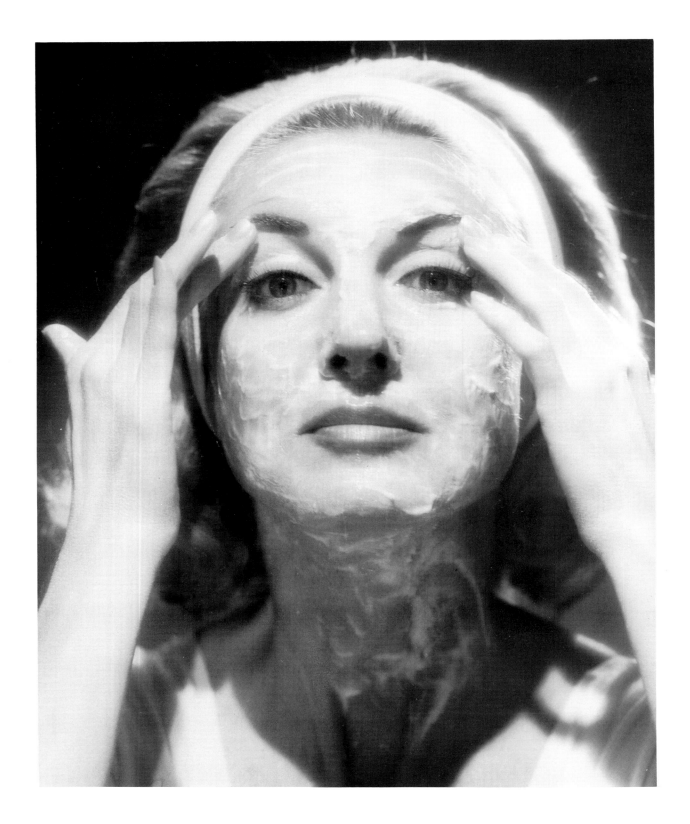

UPPER EYELIDS: While working on the upper eyelids you may frown for this part by lifting up your brows in order to tighten the muscle skin of the upper eyelid.

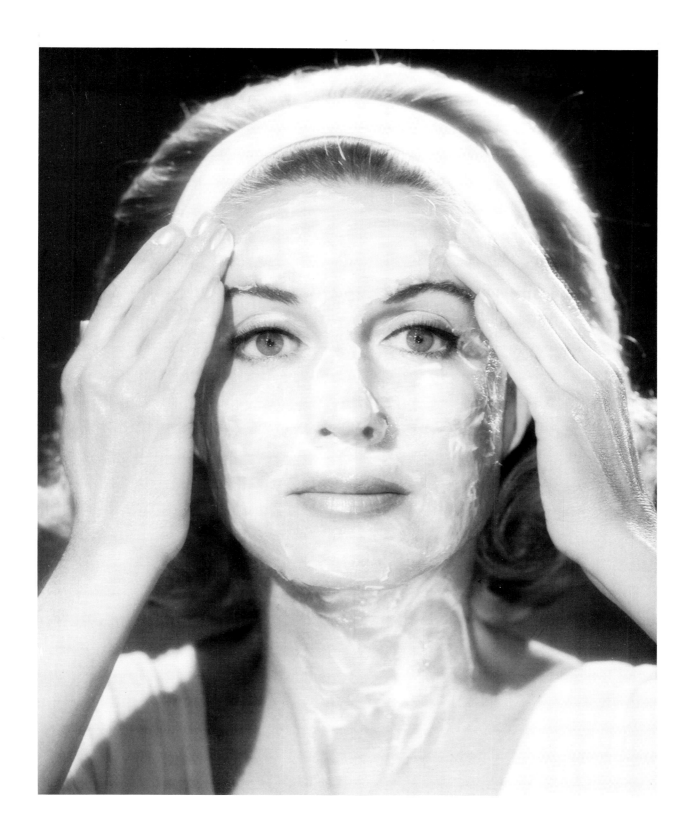

FOREHEAD: The skin of the forehead can only be held immobile by holding it with one hand against the bone underneath while working with the other hand.

By cleansing your skin in the position described and illustrated you will realize how much cleaner your skin will be compared to the results you obtain from the usual pushing around you probably give it. Those having aged, wrinkled, or creased skin will find that this method of cleansing the skin permits you to reach into those folds that have been neglected and are greatly in need of lubrication and nourishment.

Make-up applied on a tight skin will appear smoother and more even, providing the foundation was tight. Just for a moment, let us compare a loose and wrinkled skin to a deflated balloon. Now imagine that you paint over the balloon while it is deflated, then you blow it up. Examination will show that much of the surface has received no color at all. It is the same with the skin, and remember it is always the areas or tissues that need the most attention that get the least.

CHAPTER IV

Beauty Of Expression

THE POWER OF EXPRESSION

Although it is said that Mona Lisa was a beautiful woman, it was her expression - her smile - that fascinated Leonardo de Vinci who preserved her famous smile for almost 500 years. Skin quality and structural form are basic beauty assets of the face; the expression is the manager or administrator of these assets. Depending on its ability to do this job, your facial expression may increase or decrease the value of your basic state of beauty. Your facial expression creates the first impression on observers - and the first one usually is lasting. Your entire future - marriage, social happiness, and business success - may depend upon your first impression to persons you meet.

Expression is a state of mind that is transferred by actions into unspoken words that may have an irresistable power of attraction or repulsion.

ATTRACTIVE EXPRESSION: This attraction, which has a magic power - especially toward the opposite sex - is termed charm. Your beauty is increased under the management of attractive expression.

LACK OF EXPRESSION: Expressionless faces are tasteless - like food without salt. The beauty of your facial skin and form receives no benefit from this insipid management.

REPULSIVE EXPRESSION: Repelling expression is the manager that ruins the estate of beauty.

YOUR EXPRESSION LABELS YOU

No part of you is more expressive or fascinating than your face. Your mental attitude and emotional life both are illustrated in it; the quality of your personality shows in your expression. The eyes, which are called the windows of the soul, express emotions involuntarily. The voluntary tools for facial expression are muscles which are partially or completely attached to the skin and activated by subconscious or conscious will to determine the appearance of the face. The first impression a person creates is judged by the form of her or his facial features. Paintings and drawings — particularly cartoons and caricatures that allow exaggeration — introduce and tell their stories by the kind of characters being depicted by their features of expression. An expression of attention or surprise is given by raising the frontalis — which elevates the eyebrows and consequently wrinkles the forehead. If this action is exaggerated by raising the eyebrows still higher, the expression becomes one of fright or ferocity. Pulling the eyebrows together in a vertical scowl creates an expression of disapproval, scrutiny or criticism. Pulling the mouth corners down expresses skepticism or sadness. NOW YOU CAN UNDERSTAND THAT THESE FEATURES CAN DISTURB EVEN THE MOST BEAUTIFUL FACE.

HOW TO EXPRESS A BEAUTIFUL 'YOU'

The most beautiful expression is, of course, that of love and compassion. Expression reflects the inner self, where the highest interpretation of beauty is possible; for as Henry Thomas said so wisely "Beauty is not only a physical invitation to life, it is especially a spiritual confirmation of life". Beauty, in fact, does not exist outside until our awareness of it unfolds within. Beauty is a concept, created by and projected from our inner resources. Whenever you direct your thoughts inwards, you will suddenly discover that YOU are the creator of your concepts of beauty, which lie in the spiritual realm within. To acquire such a sublime asset one has to be able to love oneself, a gift accessible to everyone, simply for the asking. Prove it to yourself by practicing the following: Each night just before falling asleep simply tell yourself, **"I enjoy being me"**. Listen to these words while you repeat them a few times. Your subconscious mind will then take over and work for you. After you have practiced this simple and most effective suggestion for a while, you will, upon awakening, begin to behold in the mirror the very person whose facial expression confirms, "I enjoy being me". If we can accept and love ourselves, we can love the world.

CHAPTER V

Beauty Of Contour

THE MUSCLE STRUCTURE OF OUR FACE

The muscle flesh covering our frame-work of bones gives the body and face their shape. On our body we call it "figure", on our face we call it "contour", and it is this particular YOU that has the power to express what is termed "sex appeal" and therefore contributes the major part to our individual physical beauty appearance. Because of the skin, you are unable to see the actual muscle structure of your face. However, even from the outside you can pretty well evaluate the condition of your muscle tissues - whether they have kept their firmness or have collapsed with passing time.

By comparing pictures taken over the years, you can see how the contour of the face has changed. At the age of 2 it looked different than at our very first birthday, and with 10 years we looked much different than at the age of 20. From one day to the other our face never looks the same. Facial contour changes are so gradual that they are imperceptible by daily checks in a mirror. Those who are not alert to contour changes may ask, "What makes my face look different now?" Although contour change, skin condition, and expression are all contributing factors, it is the contour change which carries the largest part in the change of growing up and growing old.

Our muscle flesh is not a solid and fixed matter. It lives by the biological process of constantly building, shaping and changing from the beginning to the end of our physical life. The muscles are of flexible, elastic tissues, from which we build and mold their shape. The food or the nutrition which we take in is the material by which our thoughts and actions can sculpture the face to our heart's desire.

YOUTH OF CONTOUR AND ITS DECLINE

The contour of the face is determined by the condition of the muscles beneath the skin which have the function to hold the shape of its flesh and to execute our will through nerve telegraphy, since each muscle ending is connected to our brain.

A young face has an evenly formed and firm shape because the muscles are strong and elastic. However, once the biological process of growing up is completed, the face begins to change its contour enroute "down" due to gradual elongation of the muscles responding to gravity's pull. Between the ages of 21 and 40 for instance, the upper cheek muscles may have elongated as much as half an inch, and by the age of 60, as much as one inch, which means that we have one inch too much hanging over the lower part of the face. This results in hollowness in the upper cheeks below the cheek bones, fullness and flabbiness in the lower cheeks, pouches from the mouth to the chin, folds above the laugh line, drooping mouth corners and jowls. The muscles constituting the upper eyelids may elongate as much as half an inch or more between the ages of 20 and 60, causing eyebrows to shift down and upper eyelids to overlap lashes, making the eyes appear smaller. The tiny muscles constituting our lower eyelids may elongate approximately half an inch, and those muscles attached to our throat skin, as much as two inches, resulting in what is termed a "turkey neck."

The skin, of course, always follows its foundation, which is the muscle structure, givng the impression of having too much skin sagging and overlapping. Yet, it is always the underlying muscle foundation that pulls the skin along with it.

Since the cause of contour decline is muscle elongation, it stands to reason that to remedy this we have to shorten the muscle group responsible for same. The skin will always adapt to the size of its underlying foundation. All this time the aging process of the face has been diagnosed incorrectly by assuming that the fault was with the skin and that wrinkles alone portrayed age. To believe that as long as a face does not bear any lines, it has not lost its youth, is believing an old wife's tale, and so is the concept that lines are tell-tale signs of the age of a person. First, everyone knows women or men who, despite being around their seventieth year, have beautiful, wrinkle-free, tight looking "baby skin". Of course, such a skin is supported by plenty of fatty pillows, nevertheless, it is a skin free of wrinkles such as many young people wish they might have. Yet, despite the young and beautiful looking skin, the face looks like that of a person around seventy years old. Why? Because it is the form, the contour shaped by the muscle structure beneath the skin, that causes us to make a first impressional opinion of a person's age. We all agree that wrinkles and lines are unattractive in any face, whether youthful or mature. It is, however, the positioning of the muscle flesh, for instance of the cheeks and upper eyelids, by which the onlooker perceives and judges a person's age. Every tiny millimeter increase in the shifting downward of a muscle section, announces, not kindly, the sum total of birthdays. On the average, it is around the middle of the twentieth year when the first signs of muscular relaxation become visible to most persons, but the process itself has started earlier, at approximately the end of the 'teens. However, no general rule is applicable, since the maintenance of muscle tone depends on individual muscle condition which in turn depends on one's general health and nutrition as well as on the climate to which a face has been exposed. (Incidentally, protein and the Vitamin B's are essential muscle-building supplements.) Muscles that have been kept overtired, due to lack of sleep, have the tendency to collapse rapidly. An overworked or overstrained muscle will give the same symptoms of collapse as does an underactive muscle. A tired body muscle tells us through aches to relax it by sitting or lying down. A facial muscle — when tired — will not ache, it will show! We say, "You look tired." Even a baby shows tiredness in the face in the form of circles and tiny lines in the lower eyelid area, but after sufficient sleep the circles and lines disappear. In later years these circles and lines will become lasting and extensive due to tiredness and a consequent lack of circulation.

WHY DO WE HAVE TO EXERCISE OUR FACIAL MUSCLES AGAINST PROPER RESISTANCE?

Facial muscles cannot be adequately strengthened by normal activities such as blinking, smiling, eating, talking, etc., since they constitute a) involuntary movements and b) do not contract the muscles involved to their fullest capacity.

Only isometric facial excercises are of value to the facial muscles. An isometric facial exercise is possible only if a muscle or muscle group is worked against proper resistance, whereby the resistance has to be held *exactly* at the point of muscle function, thereby permitting the fullest muscle expansion (contraction) at the slowest range possible. Any other muscle movement cannot be considered an exercise but only a waste of time. Bear in mind that we move our facial muscles all day by talking, laughing, blinking, etc., and yet in every face all of those muscles collapse.

A valid facial exercise, which requires moving a designated muscle section against proper resistance as outlined in my instructions, has to show immediate results. The underlying reason for these results in the face is that a muscle can only be moved against its resistance, by its fibres shortening. The muscle tissues then are able to retain some of this shortness, at least long enough for us to evaluate the exercise performance in our mirror. The degree of mentioned results depends on the individual tissue elasticity. Shortened muscle tissues (which is our aim) provide a lift and some firmness within the exercised area. It stands to reason that results will increase in magnitude and retention ability with increase of tissue elasticity due to persistent exercising. With this knowledge you can determine instantly if you have done an exercise correctly or not.

CAN ISOMETRIC EXERCISES BE SUBSTITUTED BY A MACHINE?

The only effective remedy for shortening and firming muscle tissues is isometric exercise at the impetus of the mind. As long as an individual brain cannot be substituted by a machine, there cannot be a substitute for voluntary isometric exercises. Therapeutical electrical stimulation is used only up to the point where a muscle cannot contract voluntarily. My method of isometric facial exercises must never be combined with any facial machine regardless of what an advertisement promises. Likewise, massage or other promising manipulations do not take the place of nor do they support exercises. On the contrary, massage has been designed for the purpose of relaxing muscles. Such treatments applied to the face logically promote the collapse of our facial muscles. Therefore, any such manipulations aimed at the facial skin or muscles must be omitted, although at the time of application the face seems to respond favorably.

WHAT YOU NEED TO KNOW TO LEARN MY EXERCISES:

A. Point of Action

Like body muscles, most of the facial muscles originate at a bone. In the body, most muscles stretch over an area to connect with another bone. In the facial structure, the muscle flesh originating at a bone stretches over an area — where it constitutes a particular section of our facial contour — then attaches to the skin at which point the muscle performs its function. The point of function is important for my particular method of exercising the facial muscles.

B. Principles of my Exercises

The basic principle of my method is to keep the entire face and body relaxed and to move the designated muscle group only. To move a designated muscle group freely by its own effort, the surrounding muscles have to remain inactive and relaxed. This takes concentration and practice. Tension hardens the flesh and makes it difficult, if not impossible, to be moved. Helping or bracing the designated muscles by other muscles, relieves the "wanted ones" from doing their job and one is not helping one's face. Principle number two of my method is to move a muscle to a count. Each count is a command of the mind to the muscle to move. Please do not count to the movements but move to the count.

C. The Ultimate of Every Exercise in my Method

Every muscle or muscle group has a certain range of expansion possibility. You will find it is easier to expand a muscle in one quick movement than in several slow movements. Make a test and lift your arm up once quickly and the second time very slowly. Slow movements impose much more work on muscles than do fast movements. If, for instance, your smiling muscles have an expansion possibility of one inch and you expand (contract) this one inch in ten-step-movements, the smiling muscles have worked ten times as hard as if they had taken the one inch in one step. This being so, we start out expanding the designated muscle section in one full movement, which is the easiest way. Once you have learned this you then should divide the full expansion in two even movements. After this lesson try for three even movements. And so you work yourself up to the minimum steps which are prescribed for each exercise and preliminary practice.

D. The Difference Between Moving and TENSING A MUSCLE

MOVING: Muscle movements shorten muscle tissues, because a muscle can only be moved by its fibers tightening up. Example: Let your arms hang down. Now very slowly raise your arms — elbows straight — and observe the work imposed on the muscles in moving the arms. Take note that the slower you move the more the muscles have to work. Remember this for your facial exercises.

TENSING: Contrary to muscle movements, muscle tension merely hardens the tissues and hinders same from moving. Example: Let your arms hang down and increasingly flex your fist. Note that you do not move any muscles but that you merely tense same up which causes the muscles to harden.

E. The Importance of Breathing When We Exercise

Concentration so necessary for the facial exercises can be accomplished only if the brain tissues are supplied with sufficient amounts of oxygen. Therefore, deep and frequent breathing during exercising is of great importance. Insufficient breathing causes muscular tension which, of course hardens the muscle flesh making it difficult or even impossible to move. The brain itself requires at least twenty percent of the oxygen from the body's circulating blood. Do not forget that we also need oxygen for the muscle building process desired through our exercises.

F. Purpose of Preliminary Practice

The purpose of the preliminary practice is:
a) to gain awareness of the isolated muscle group on which we wish to work,
b) to learn to move the isolated muscle group at its point of action freely, by itself, without help from other muscles.
c) to bring the isolated muscle group under the control of our mind by moving the muscle to a count.

G. Principles of Resistance

Holding a rubber band on one end enables us to expand it. When we hold a muscle on one end, we too, can expand its elastic fibers very slowly and extensively which is necessary for the chemical process to take place.

Two principles of resistance are implied in these exercises. For expression muscles, the needed resistance is set up by pressing the skin against the nearest bone. The exercise is then — by will power — to move the muscles against the resistance. To the other muscles, resistance is given by grasping them at the point of action between the fingers or with Face-Ex and then — by will power — moving the muscles at their point of action against the resistance. The resistance must always be kept steady and must not be allowed to move during an exercise.

After you have completed an exercise, check for results, and also for the finger marks on your face to see whether the resistance was correctly and evenly applied.

RECOMMENDED SKIN CARE WHEN APPLYING MY EXERCISES

Some of my exercises call for a protective coating which we obtain from my Exercise Creme. The purpose of my Exercise Creme in particular is to protect the superficial layers of the epidermis from creasing where it cannot be avoided. My Exercise Creme has been designed to give you adequate protection. The cream must be applied thickly and has to cover all of the area around your eyes that may crease when smiling up. Otherwise, the facial skin must be kept dry and free of any application during exercising. Should you detect other lines in your face while exercising, disqualify that particular exercise; it indicates tension or insufficient resistance. When doing EXERCISE No. 1, No. 1-B, or No. 2 it is recommended to apply several drops of Senta Maria Rungé's Tears of Venus (Vita-Ex) Throat Oil to the neck-muscle-skin.

To obtain the best benefits from applying my method it is important that you prepare your skin properly for the exercises

1. BY PROVIDING THE SKIN'S TISSUES WITH THE PLIABILITY NECESSARY FOR THE EXERCISES.

2. BY DEEP CLEANSING ITS SUPERFICIAL LAYERS.

All of these preparatory qualifications are built into Senta Maria Runge's CREAM FOR CLEANSING which has been especially formulated for this purpose.

Step A.   Thoroughly cleanse your skin of face and neck with Senta Maria Runge's ESPECIALLY FORMULATED CREAM FOR CLEANSING. Follow with a lukewarm to warm water rinse. Towel dry your cleansed skin.

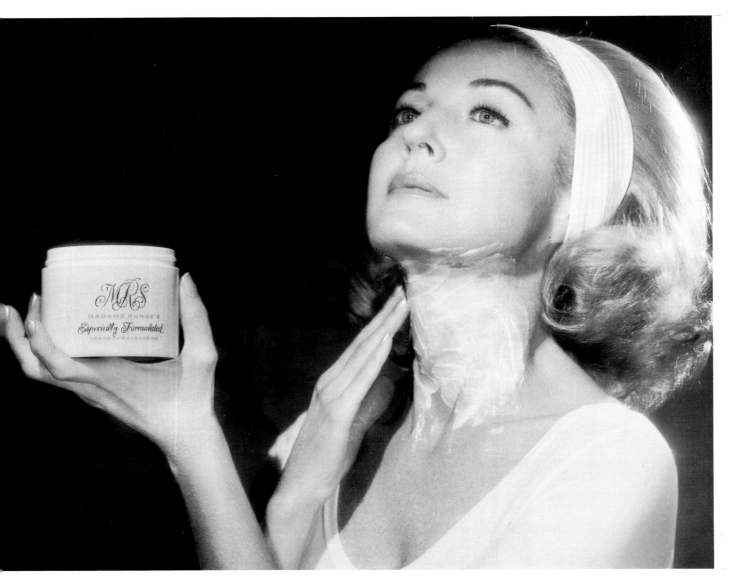

Step B.   After the exercises apply a cold water rinse consisting of ten generous splashes of cold soft water. Water may be softened by adding one heaping teaspoon of baking soda or boric acid to a sinkful of water.

EXERCISE PROCEDURE

A.   First locate the particular muscle group responsible for the contour fault you wish to correct. Do this by comparing the analysis chart with your mirrored picture and the muscle face.

B.   With soft eyebrow pencil draw on the face the location of the muscle group you wish to work on, as it is marked on the photo.

C.   First learn the PRELIMINARY PRACTICE.

D.   Once you have perfected the PRELIMINARY PRACTICE proceed with the isometric exercise. As soon as you are able to apply the isometric exercise, omit its PRELIMINARY PRACTICE.

TOOLS RECOMMENDED FOR EXERCISING

a) Senta Maria Runge's ESPECIALLY FORMULATED CREAM FOR CLEANSING
b) Senta Maria Runge's EXERCISE CREMÉ
c) Senta Maria Runge's TEARS OF VENUS Throat Oil when exercising neck or jowl bags.
d) a flexible mirror to stand in front of you
e) soft tissue napkins cut in approximately 1½ inch squares
f) soft eyebrow pencil
g) cosmetic gloves or other thin cotton gloves
h) scowl object when exercising vertical lines between the brows.

EXERCISE RULES

1. READ THIS BOOK FROM THE BEGINNING TO THE END BEFORE ATTEMPTING YOUR FIRST EXERCISE.

2. RESULTS ARE GUARANTEED, HOWEVER, ONLY IF THE INSTRUCTIONS ARE APPLIED **VERBATIM** ON A STEP-BY-STEP BASIS.

3. Every time read the instruction to the exercise you are about to apply and follow the instructions step by step.

4. If the position of your hands is incorrect, place them in the correct position after removing them completely from the face; do not move them on the skin around your eyes.

5. After one exercise is completed, remove your hands or object from your face, look at the results, then replace your hands for the next exercise application.

6. Breathe deeply and frequently.

7. After expansion, return the muscles involved under control, preferably to the number of counts given with each exercise.

8. When working a muscle against resistance, maintain even resistance. Never release resistance until muscles have returned to their starting position. Do not permit resistance to slip and if it has slipped, do not continue the exercise.

A NOTE TO MY READERS:

Please do not inquire about personal instructions. As I have stated on page 39, I closed my studio in order to dedicate my time to research. From the many testimonials I have received from around the world I know that the exercises, as set forth in this book, can be applied successfully. The degree of benefit one will achieve, depends entirely on how conscientiously my rejuvenation program and particularly my exercise instructions are followed.

CAN THE SKIN BE STRETCHED WITH THESE EXERCISES?

Facial exercises contribute immensely to the maintenance and rehabilitation of skin elasticity. Like facial muscles, the elastic fibers of our Corum need to be worked and challenged. The only possible correct way to work the elastic tissues of the skin is through expanding it by the underlying muscles. In this process, the skin is expanded only it its natural make-up and therefore cannot be overexpanded. Pushing and pulling the skin by hands stretches the skin.

The vitality or collapse of the skin depends also on circulation which facial exercises supply to the skin. This is the reason why the facial skin takes on a healthy glow from my exercises.

WORKING EXAMPLE AND TIPS FOR ISOMETRIC FACIAL EXERCISES (Cheeks) see pages 129 - 133

    a. Look into mirror and emphasize with eyebrow pencil the point of action necessary for the purpose of placing the resistance. If required, apply Senta Maria Runge's Exercise Cremé around your eyes.

    b. Position resistance precise and firm.

c. Breathe deeply - relax and close your eyes for concentration. In your mind, try to feel the muscle-flesh-skin which is held in resistance. Since it is your mind that has to move the muscle-flesh-skin, it is necessary that your mind first feels those muscles. Touching with your finger the skin at the point of resistance, sometimes assists our mind to feel the proper place.

d. Once your mind has a definite feeling of the particular muscle-flesh in resistance, check once more that you have not tensed up anywhere on face or body, - then count "o n e" and make your first attempt to move the muscle-flesh-skin out of the resistance. The resistance of course must remain immobile. By doing so you have expanded the designated muscle tissues. (Think of a rubber band.) Hold this expanded muscle position while you breathe deeply.

e. Concentrate again on "feeling" the muscle-flesh-skin at the point of resistance (for better concentration you may close your eyes). Once you "feel" the point of action which is held in resistance, count " t w o " and make another attempt to move the muscle-flesh-skin out of your immobile resistance. This action of course will extend the already existing muscle expansion. Breathe deeply - and concentrate for the next expansion step. Proceed in this fashion as long as your concentration power lasts, because forcing the issue promotes instant tension which hardens the flesh.

The effort imposed on the working muscles cause them to quiver, not only when being moved but also while the expanded position is held. Make an honest check that no other muscles quiver from working!! - Only the wanted ones!

66

f. The same procedure applies to the returning of the muscles.

    1.   Concentrate to feel the particular muscle-flesh-skin involved. Breathe.

    2.   Count and return muscle-flesh-skin one step at a time toward the resistance. (Again think of a rubberband.) Resistance remains immobile until no more muscle expansion exists.

g. Check for improvement, since only result producing exercises are valid. In case you are not sure whether or not you see results, disqualify the exercise and be assured that you will notice results if you deserve them! Re-read to find out what you did incorrect. Assuming the placement of your resistance was correct, you

    a)   either have not held the resistance immobile but went along with the muscle movement or

    b)   you tensed up with other muscles. For this keep close check on the jaw, forehead, neck or the muscles next to your resistance.

FACIAL CONTOURS IN NEED FOR
A NEW LEASE ON YOUTH

Having purchased this book and quickly glanced through it will perhaps stimulate enough enthusiasm in you for making a vow to "immediately learn all the exercises contained in this book and to do them faithfully every day". Based on my experiences with clientele I know that those thoughts and self promises are all normal, but I also know that they are rarely being followed through because of unforseen interruptions in our daily schedule and a lack of time.

In order to correct a contour fault through the process of shortening the muscles and restoring the tone, one has to apply to those muscles at fault a program of three result producing exercises in succession once a day six days a week. (Only result producing exercises count.) Also, a contour fault may be eliminated in a relatively short time, however it usually takes from three to four months to restore sufficient tone to the muscles, for them to hold the acquired condition without having to continuously exercise every day.

The actual application of everyone of my exercises takes less than one minute. However, the time necessary to relax and concentrate to move the desired muscle-flesh takes longer than the actual exercise. The benefit from everyone of the exercises depends on the exactness of its application. Quality cannot be substituted by quantity.

Since our concentration power and time for exercising is limited and the ultimate result from my facial exercises depends upon precision and persistency of application, I recommend you learn only one or two isometric exercises at a time. Once you have mastered an isometric exercise, add another one to your program. Practice your exercise(s) in an undisturbed atmosphere every day and set enough time aside so not to feel rushed. Most people seem to have their best concentration ability in the mornings after they have rested. Of course when you have to meet your job early in the morning you will find your time in the evenings more appropriate for relaxing and concentrating. Fresh air and deep breathing helps to relax and to concentrate. Many of you will require more time to learn to relax and to concentrate, than to actually lift your face with the exercises. Any coordination between mind and muscles - whether it is playing an instrument or a sport - requires concentration and persistent practice.

Whenever one wishes to correct a contour fault, one must exercise six days in succession and then permit the muscles one day of rest. You will witness with your own eyes that the muscles do respond best the day after they have rested.

Once you have shortened the desired muscle-flesh sufficiently — which is indicated by the disappearance of the contour fault — and restored adequate muscle tone, I suggest you observe how well the acquired correction holds and design your own exercise program in consideration of this. Perhaps twice or three times a week will be sufficient to maintain the condition, depending on your health, general activity and age, but you should always perform a minimum of three to four result producing exercises in succession on each desired muscle group.

HOW TO LIFT YOUR FACE
WITH A 10-MINUTE-A-DAY PROGRAM

After you have carefully read and fully comprehended the content of the book up to and including page 80, begin your program by investing 10 minutes daily, six days a week, into practicing only one exercise until perfection. I suggest for your first exercise, No. 6 for the upper cheeks, because the muscles involved in this exercise control about half the actual area of the face, consequently producing the biggest lift in everyone's face; also it serves as a classical sample exercise for all others.

At first you should study and practice at complete leisure the Preliminary to Exercise No. 6, step by step. **Do not proceed to the consequent step unless you have mastered the prior one completely.** Follow the instructions as conscientiously as they were outlined. Once you are ready for the Isometric to Exercise No. 6, be sure and incorporate into your practice every step of the Working Example on pages 56-67. Bear in mind that you must see instant results from every isometric performance, as indicated on page 131. If no results are visible, compare what you have done with the instructions to locate your error. There is absolutely no reason to be afraid of increasing your problem unless you continue to do the same adverse result producing mistake over a period of time.

Once you have learned the upper cheek exercise to the point that you obtain results from every application, you will notice that the actual exercise applications (muscle movements) do not require much more than a minute. At this point I suggest you add another exercise to your program, preferably Exercise No. 11 for lifting upper eyelids. Your experience in learning the upper cheek exercise will enable you to master the new exercise by investing only eight minutes daily in practicing and perfecting same. Once you have conquered your second exercise, you may add a third one. However, if the time you have to yourself is rather limited, it is best to exercise only the upper cheeks and upper eyelids, since those two muscle sections usually sag first and portray the indignity of aging more than the rest of the face combined.

FOR THE YOUNG FACES I advise as preventive measures Exercise for Posture Correction on page 96, six days a week, and Exercise No. 6 for the Upper Cheeks, two days a week. Set aside two regular days as Mondays and Thursdays, or Tuesdays and Fridays, and exercise three times in succession. Only a result producing performance is considered an exercise, since only those benefit the muscles. Therefore, learn to apply your facial exercises precisely as instructed. The results you will see from preventive measures are a fresher and firmer look. As the years progress, and your body's general circulation slows down, you may need to increase your facial exercise program. This should not be done by increasing the frequency of application, but by adding more days to your program. In conjunction with the other suggestions in this book, the acquired knowledge and technique will enable you to always keep your face in a firm and youthful shape.

EXPRESSION LINES AND THEIR CORRECTION

Certain facial muscles are called expression muscles because we use them to express our emotions. The expression muscles which are partially or fully attached to the skin, are subject to our conscious or subconscious actions of expression. Unlike other mucles, expression muscles do not collapse in the form of lines because of inadequate activity. Expression lines are muscles which have formed into lines by the habit of holding them for too long a period of time in the position.

Expression lines are not an adjunct of aging — young people can have them also. The extent to which those lines may be etched on the face, largely depends upon ones age, since the degree of muscle and skin elasticity is a determining factor.

The best remedy for expression lines of course is prevention, because those lines will never appear unless they are forced to appear. If you have the habit of forming lines into your face, it has to be broken for preventive as well as corrective purposes, the latter is an adjunct to the necessary corrective exercise.

GAINING MUSCLE CONTROL

Muscle control of your body gives you grace; in our cosmetic law for the face, it is the number one item. No matter along what line a habit is — smoking, drinking, overeating or frowning — one really has to work at it in order to break it. Breaking a habit requires conscious effort and will power. The habit of frowning, like other habits, is a subconscious action. To bring the muscles involved under control, you must first call them into your conscious mind. To accomplish this, one must practice frowning consciously and very slowly in front of a mirror, two or three times daily. At first frown as much as you can at once by moving the eyebrows up. The second time divide your "frown" into two even muscle movements done by the brows. First count, then move the muscles to your count. The third time divide your frown into three even movements. In this fashion practice disciplining your muscles until you can frown in ten even steps and return those muscles in ten even steps. It is essential that you permit the muscles to move only to your count, since the counting is used as a signal from your conscious mind. Do this until you are aware of this particular muscle movement (frowning) without looking into the mirror. Seeing yourself in your mirrored image frowning as others see you, may also help you to strengthen your will power to break this habit. Frowning becomes in most cases a muscular tension. I have learned of many cases where the person was unable to relax the forehead muscles, although he or she was aware that the forehead was tensed. I also have learned from some categorical frowners that they had no awareness of their forehead being tensed or relaxed. Muscles do relax under warmth, and if you are aware of your forehead tension, place your hand on the forehead and the muscles will relax. This applies also to the scowl line(s) (vertical lines) between the brows.

Do you scowl or frown in your sleep? Then apply frownies (or perhaps even scotch tape will do) over the area you move when you scowl or frown.

Pursing the lips when eating, drinking (smoking) or talking is an ugly habit which causes the very unattractive lines in the upper and lower lip. I have seen women and men under thirty with a lip of a fifty-year-old person brought upon by the before-mentioned habits. Should you belong to this category, then you may correct the condition by practicing breaking the habit through re-training your lip muscles. First look into the mirror and practice the wrong way.

Wrong way: Take a fork or a glass, or if you smoke, a cigarette, and slowly put in into your mouth whereby you purse your lips. Don't faint! Notice that pursing the lips is a muscular movement whereby the middle part of the upper lip is lifted up and the mouth corners consequently drawn inward.

Right way: The correction is being made by reversing the muscular movements. Eat, drink or speak by consistently keeping the middle part of the upper lip lower down than the rest of the upper lip. The mouth corners should give you the feeling that they are slightly turned up.

HOW MUCH CAN ONE EXPECT
FROM FACE LIFTING BY EXERCISE

The acquired knowledge and technique of the exercises contained in this book will enable you to always keep your facial contour in a firm and youthful shape. Or as a plastic surgeon wrote in his book, "If you do proper facial exercises, then you will not be interested in the chapter 'Surgical Face Lifting.'"

It is never too late to start. Keep in mind that the mechanical and chemical process of our pliable muscle tissues causes them to constantly form and shape from the beginning to the end of their existence. So—why not form them into a youthful and attractive shape? I have letters of evidence regarding results from my exercises from women at the age of 82. Of course, results at this age are considerably more limited compared to the possibilities of earlier years. However, it is always worthwhile to work toward looking ten to twenty years younger and more attractive at any age.

If my exercises are applied as instructed, the results are nothing short of amazing at any age. Most of my exercises — if done correctly — produce instantaneous results, especially in areas where the muscles are attached to the skin as on the forehead, underneath the eyes, and in the crow's feet area. But we also get marvelous results on parts where the muscles lie deeper, as in the cheeks and jowls, by a good and properly applied resistance exercise which produces an immediate lift. I have proven these statements on my television program "FACE LIFTING BY EXERCISE" from 1961 until 1963, which was broadcasted in Hollywood live and for other cities in the United States on Kinescope film. None of my models knew any more, and perhaps even less, than you know about facial resistance exercises. Each one had to learn the exercises right in front of the camera, which made the situation exciting for everyone. Each exercise takes only about twenty to thirty seconds and has to be repeated three times in succession. With this technique the models removed wrinkles from underneath the eyes, the crow's feet, scowl and frown lines in just a few minutes and right in front of the camera. It is understandable that the results will not last forever, and that one has to persistently exercise in this manner six days a week until the muscle has enough tone to completely hold its acquired condition. So, if we planned not to cover an already started exercise in the next program, the models and the audience were told to do those by themselves.

I am certain that you, too, have discovered that, given two ways of doing a thing, our perhaps perverse natures make us choose the wrong or difficult way! And this, too, was an exciting part of our daily performance. The best way (not always the easiest though) is to learn and find out through making mistakes. Since correctly applied resistance exercises have the power to tighten up a muscle so amazingly fast, it stands to reason that incorrect performance produces negative results. Maybe a muscle has not been held in the right position or the resistance has not been held firmly enough, or a muscle slipped or was relaxed too quickly. Whatever it was, the models had to find out or I pointed it out to them — and with the next exercise, done properly, the damage was immediately corrected. Sometimes it also happened that after an exercise the model's face was lopsided for awhile, maybe one cheek or one mouth corner higher than the other; that was because the exercise was performed better on one side than on the other. Every face has a weaker and a stronger side, and since it is easier to work with stronger muscles, the results there will show faster and better. After working with one model for four months, conplimentary letters poured in, claiming that the model looked about twenty years younger. This is my answer to the question

"HOW MUCH CAN ONE EXPECT FROM MY FACIAL EX-ERCISES?" On the last pages of this book you will find excerpts from letters which answer this question from persons who participated in my program right in front of their television sets at home.

Depending on muscle and skin condition, all of the mentioned contour faults in this book can be corrected completely or at the very least, greatly improved. Benefits from the exercises, of course, depend on precision of application. Most of my isometric exercises produce instant visible results. In fact after every exercise you must see results, because if you do not see results, it tells you that you have done something incorrectly; you must discover what it is you did or did not do — and then correct your error. Age is no excuse or exception for not obtaining instant results. My isometric facial exercises comprise a scientific formula for an instant shortening of facial muscles. It is the accrued day-by-day results that assure you the Facelift!

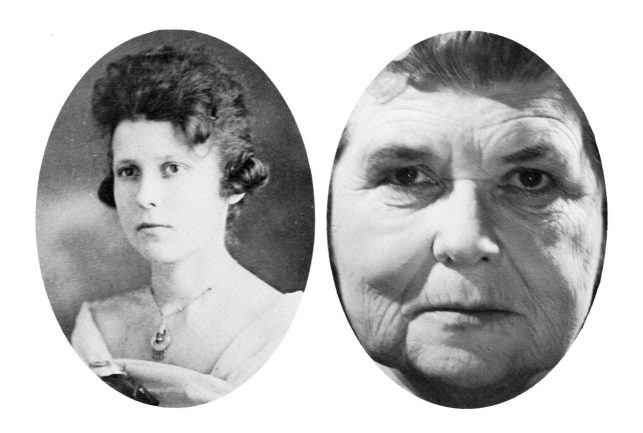

How The Years Sneak Up On Us

Ella, at her time of youth had many natural beauty assets given to her by Nature. So shows not only her picture of many years ago, but also the basic structure of her mature face. Gravity's pull over many years has now perfected a matron's face.

Many of you will see the collapse of Ella's face as an entirety, whereas I divided it into sections according to the muscle structure of the face.

ANALYSIS CHART:

AREA:	EXERCISE:
No. 1	Neck
No. 2	Jowls
No. 3	Back of Cheeks and Temples
No. 4	Lower Cheeks
No. 5	Pouch
No. 6	Upper Cheeks
No. 7	Upper Lip
No. 8	Lower Lip and Chin
No. 9	Horizontal Lines on Forehead
No. 10	Vertical Lines on Forehead
No. 11	Upper Eyelids
No. 12	Lower Eyelids
No. 13	Crow's feet
No. 15	Bridge of Nose

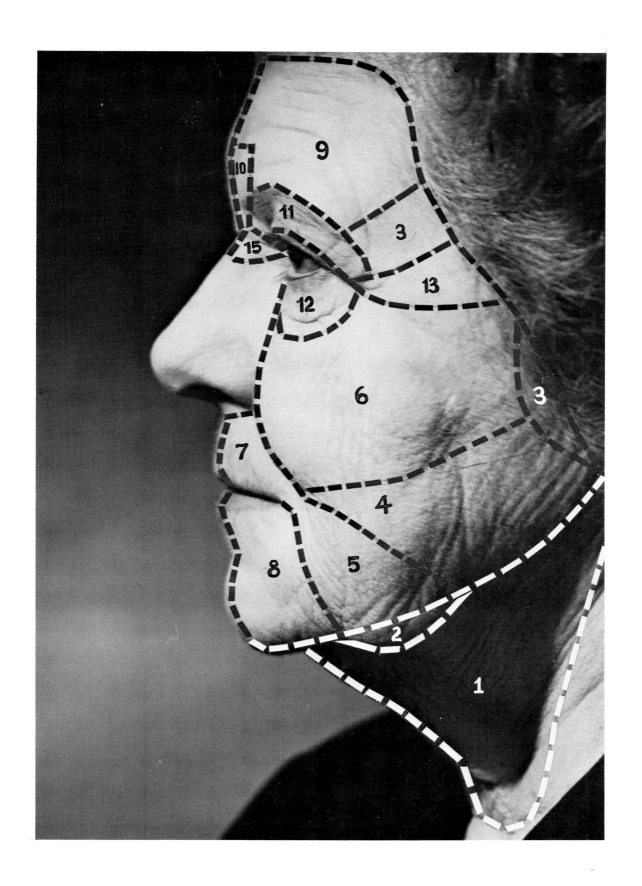

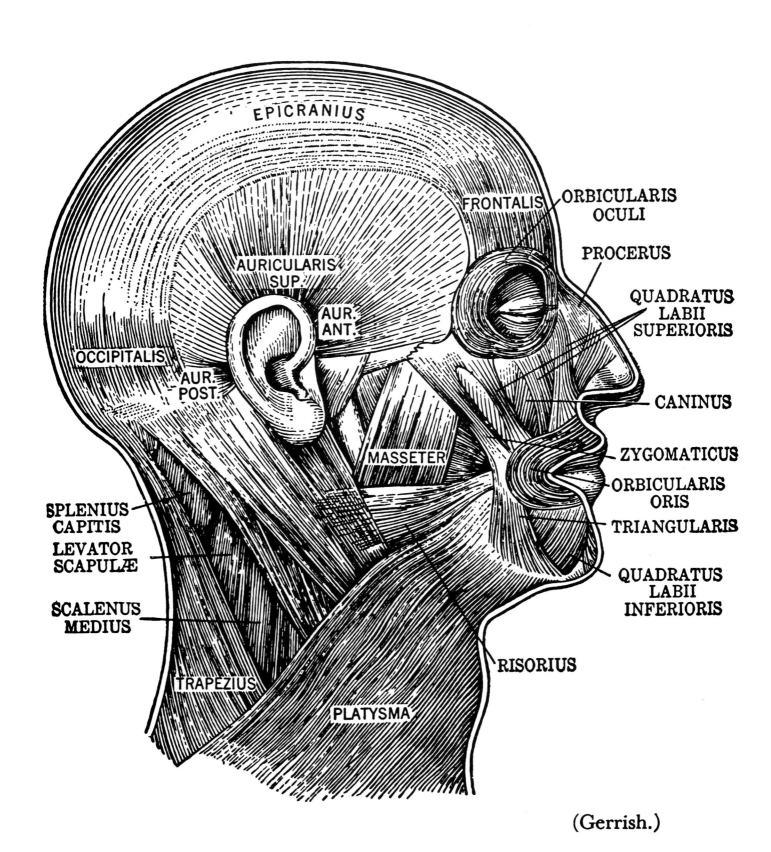

EPICRANIUS

FRONTALIS

ORBICULARIS OCULI

PROCERUS

QUADRATUS LABII SUPERIORIS

AURICULARIS SUP.

AUR. ANT.

OCCIPITALIS

AUR. POST.

CANINUS

MASSETER

ZYGOMATICUS

ORBICULARIS ORIS

SPLENIUS CAPITIS

TRIANGULARIS

LEVATOR SCAPULÆ

QUADRATUS LABII INFERIORIS

SCALENUS MEDIUS

RISORIUS

TRAPEZIUS

PLATYSMA

(Gerrish.)

80

FACE LIFTING
BY EXERCISE

by SENTA MARIA RUNGÉ

Corrective Neck—Exercises

"Loose skin will regain its firmness with the muscles since the skin is only as firm as the muscle flesh structure beneath it."

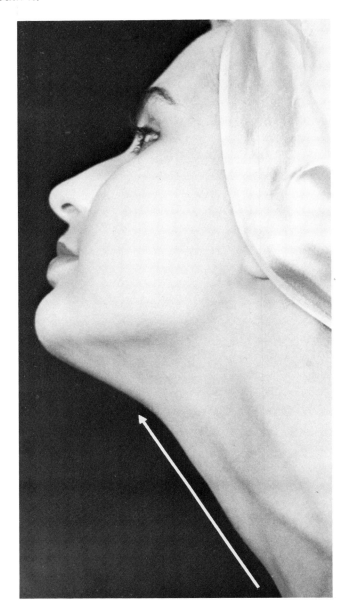

Due to the collapse of various muscle groups constituting the front part of our neck, we encounter various undesirable symptoms in this area because of decreasing muscle tone and consequent elongation of those muscles involved.

Choose the appropriate exercise to eliminate your personal problem(s).

ENCOURAGEMENT: Once a popular movie actress, whose aging neck was threatening her career, started applying my Resistance Neck Exercise and after one week exclaimed jubilantly, "My neck hasn't looked this good in fifteen years!"

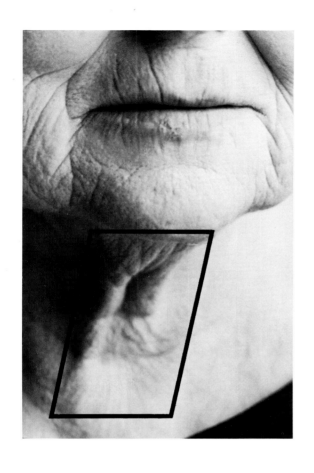

For Eliminating Vertical Cords (Turkey Neck).

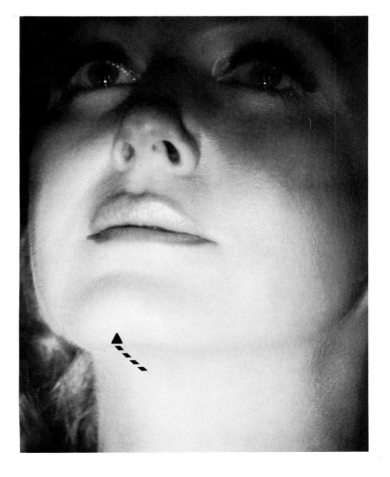

to isolate and to gain awareness of the neck muscles causing protruding cords.

---Sitting or standing position — look into mirror.

a) With eyebrow pencil draw line at the center of chin bone starting about ½-¾ inches under the chin bone.

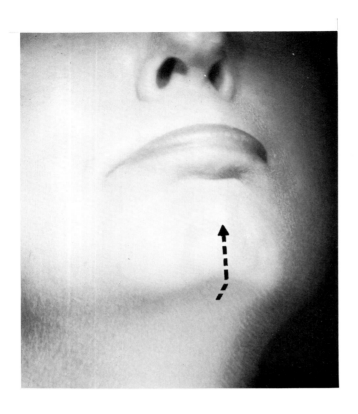

b) Relaxed, keep teeth together — lower teeth in back of upper teeth (which is the position of a normal bite).

c) In this position now practice moving the pencil line o v e r your chin bone which you do by moving the underneath lying muscle-skin. Range of this muscle movement is approximately ½ - ¾ inch. A dab of cream on your lips may be helpful so as not to hinder the lips from moving.

d) Consciously and gradually return the pencil line to starting position by returning the muscle skin.

Purpose: Moving designated muscles freely without tension or help by surrounding muscles.

Note: This is very easy to do if you keep your chin relaxed and concentrate. Mouth corners do not help but should remain immobile!

Refer: Page (58) — AIM: 10 steps, return in 10 steps.

Frequency: As often as you may wish until you have conquered the AIM.

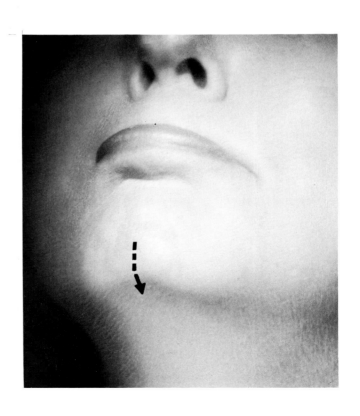

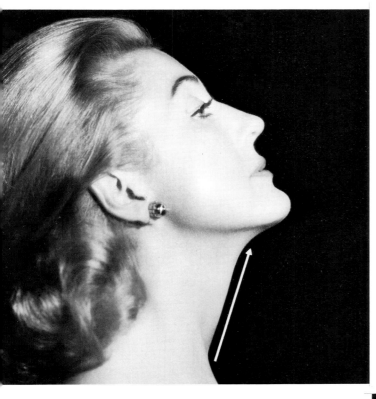

ISOMETRIC EXERCISE:

- - - Do not attempt unless PRE-LIMINARY PRACTICE HAS BEEN MASTERED.

- - - Draw line at center of chin bone as before.

- - - Apply several drops of Senta Maria Runge's VITA-EX throat oil on the skin of your front neck.

- - - Hold mirror in your hand.

Step 1. Keep shoulders straight and do not move shoulders while you jut chin forward and then upward. Entire front neck must be taut. Compare with picture.

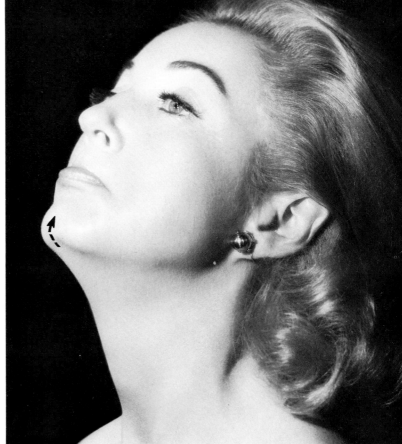

Step 2. Keep teeth relaxed together — lower teeth in back of upper teeth.

Step 3. In this position now move the pencil line o v e r your chin bone as you have practiced before.

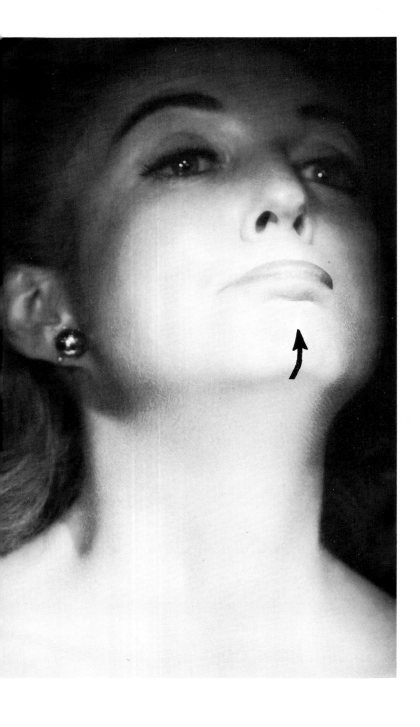

Step 4. Push the <u>tip</u> of the tongue against the inside of lower front teeth (gum line) increasing pressure with the tip of tongue for 6 gradual and definite steps.

Step 5. Consciously and gradually return <u>tip</u> of tongue, then the chin muscles (pencil line) and last the head to starting position.

Purpose: Expanding designated muscles freely without tension or help by surrounding muscles — against resistance.

Note: If done correctly, muscle-skin around chin bone will quiver when being moved. If it does not quiver, check for tension and relax it.

Refer: Page (58) — AIM: 15 steps, return in 10 steps.

Frequency: Once a day 3 times in succession.

Results: Instantly after applying 10-step-movements around chin.

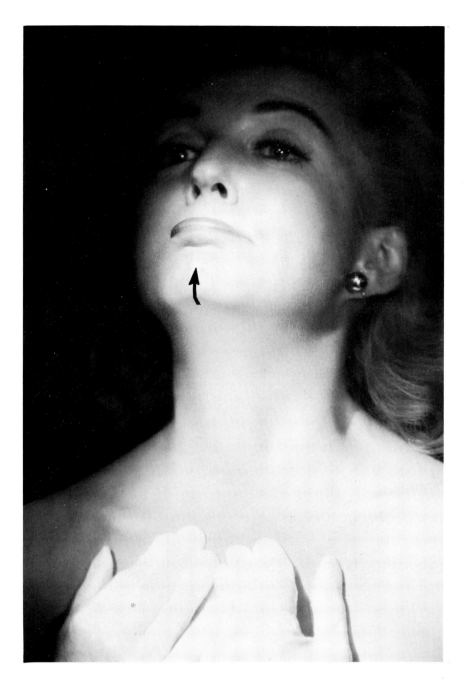

SUGGESTION:

Once you have mastered moving the muscle-skin around chin bone for ten counts, then concentrate mostly on moving the weaker side of your neck by trying to concentrate moving the more protruding cord upward and around chin bone. Do this without strain but simply by concentration.

After you have learned the above exercise, you may increase the benefits from exercising by applying additional resistance which you create by holding skin firmly against edge of bone (with your fingers).

EXERCISE NO. 1-A

ISOMETRIC
EXERCISE:

For Firming Flabby Muscles Under The Chin (Double Chin).

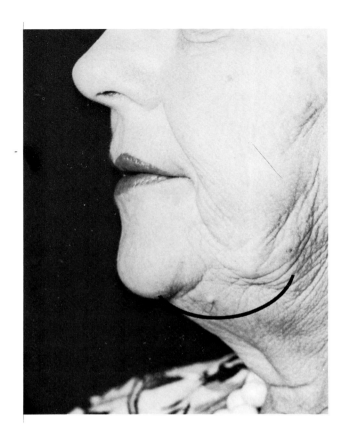

Step 1. Lift chin slightly upward;

Step 2. With flat point of index and middle fingers press against indentation (hollow) formed by the two upper nodules of the larynx located at the curve from chin to neck. Do not be concerned in the beginning as to the precise location of pressure which you will discover through practice. Regard finger pressure as the resistance against the working muscles.

Step 3. Now press your back teeth firmly together* and while maintaining this position,

Step 4. press the tip of your tongue against the inside of lower front teeth (gum line) increasing pressure with the tip of tongue** in 10 or more gradual and definite steps.

Step 5. Hold end position of pressure for 6 seconds (count slowly to six).

Step 6. Release muscle work for 10 gradual steps.

Step 7. Remove finger resistance.

Repeat 2-3 more times.

Results: Visible in approximately one week.

Note:
 *) if resistance is kept at the right place you will feel the muscles pushing against your finger resistance.

 **) For each increase of pressure with tip of tongue you will sense a stronger push against your resistance.

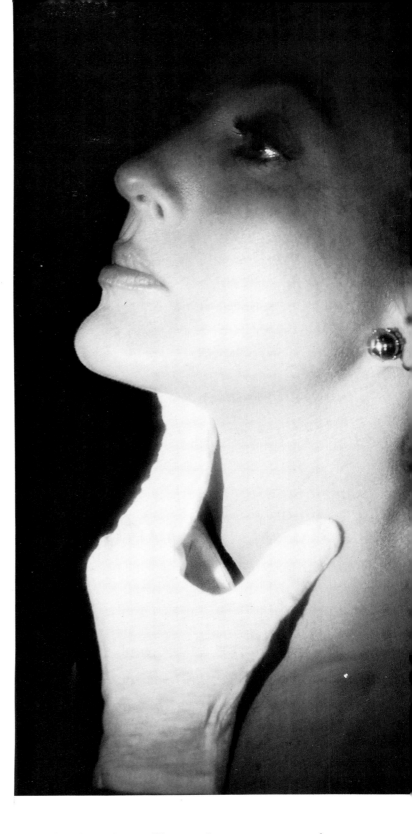

Suggestion: Since the pressure of the finger tips against resistance may be felt unpleasantly and also may slip, it is advisable to cushion finger tips with cotton.

EXERCISE NO. 1-B

For Firming & Building Up A Flabby & Scrawney Lower Neck

(General Neck Exercise)

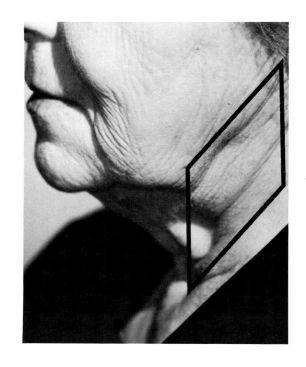

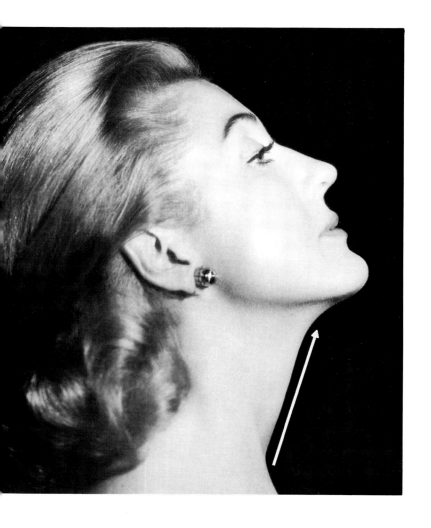

- - - Sitting or standing position — look into mirror.

- - - Apply several drops of Senta Maria Runge's VITA-EX throat oil on the skin of your front neck.

Step 1. Assume position in picture by moving chin upward. Entire front neck must feel taut.

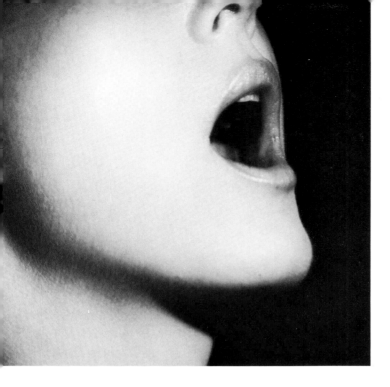

Step 2. Drop jaw down as far as possible.

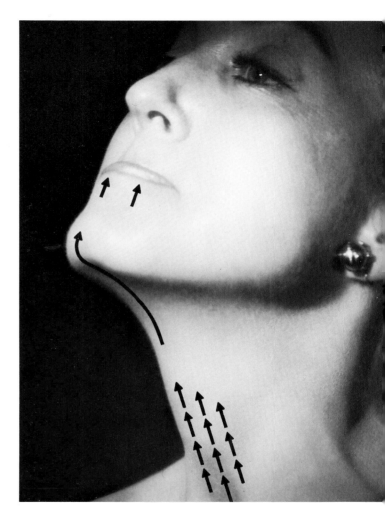

Step 3. Move jaw slightly forward and move it gradually up while concentrating on pulling the muscles in the neck from the collar bone upward. Move lower teeth and lip over the upper teeth and lip.

Step 4. While lower teeth and lip are held over the upper lip and teeth, smile with mouth corners backward and upward and hold this position for 6 seconds with concentration on a good muscle pull around and over the jaw bone.

Step 5. Slowly bring jaw down and repeat 3-4 more times.

Results: Visible in approximately one week.

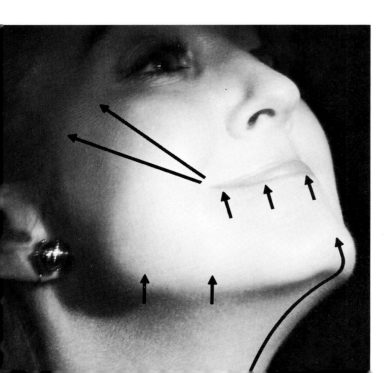

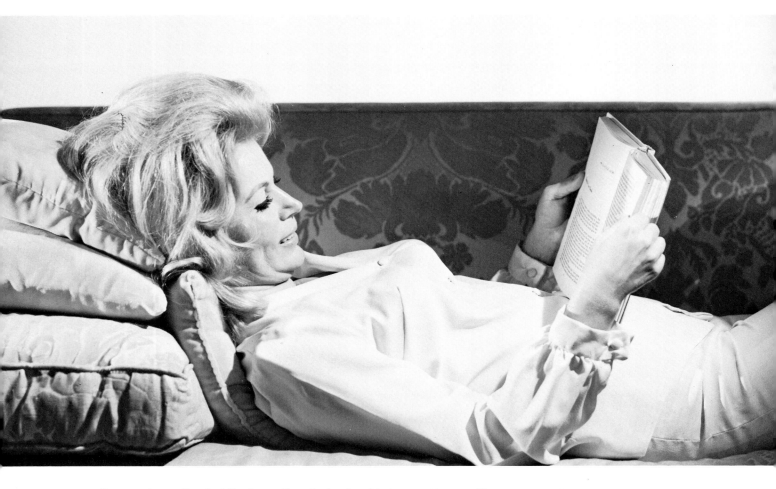

Do you have the habit of reading in bed, with two or three pillows beneath your head? — Get rid of the pillows for the sake of your neck and lower cheeks!

ADDITIONAL SUGGESTIONS FOR THE IMPROVEMENT OF THE NECK

DOUBLE CHINS. It is necessary to distinguish between two types of double chins: One which is caused by collapsed muscles beneath the skin of the neck and the other by incorrect head and body posture. As an average, people under twenty years of age do not have flaccid neck muscles to the point that they would show a double chin, but many young people do show a double chin and/or a short chin line because of the way they hold the head and body when they sit, stand and walk. This double chin will disappear immediately, if the posture is corrected. Quite frequently I have young actors and actresses visit me at my Hollywood Salon worried lest his or her double chin endanger or interfer with a movie career. In every such case it takes me no longer than a minute to remove the double chin. Secret? "Posture correction"

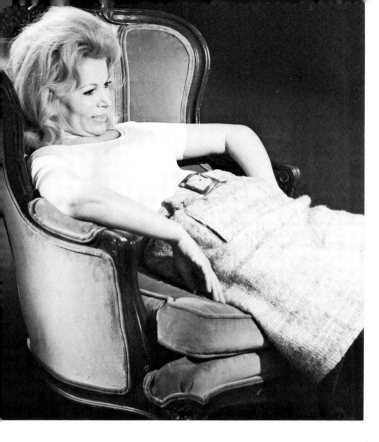

FIND OUT THE DIFFERENCE:

Sitting: If when you sit in an easy chair or on a couch your buttocks are on the front edge and your back is resting against the back of the furniture, you will show a double chin associated with deep lines in your neck. As you change this position by sliding your buttocks back, trying to sit tall, holding your torso straight, pulling the abdominal muscles in, shoulder blades back and down, chin somewhat forward but level, your neck will be slenderized and double chin(s) with associated lines will disappear.

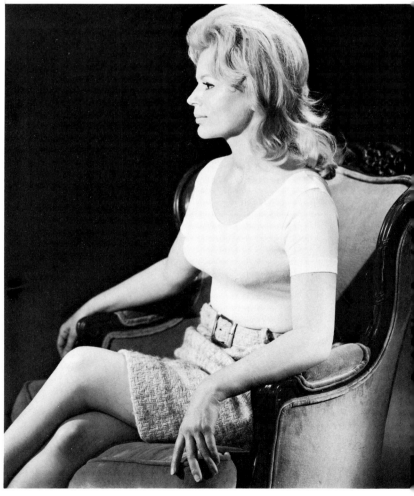

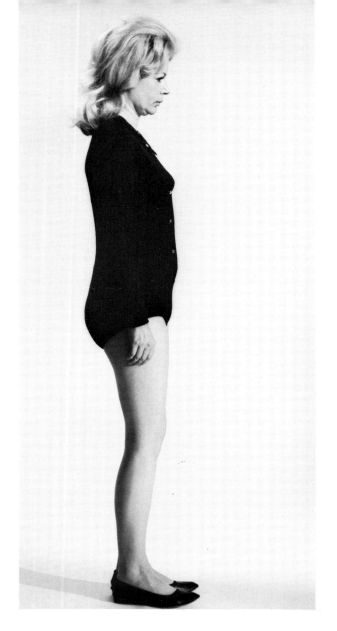

Standing: If when you stand you put the weight of your body on the heels of your feet, your neck will appear thick and lined and a double chin will be evident. As you balance your weight on the balls of your feet, especially on the joints of the big toes, shoulder blades back and down, chin somewhat forward but level, you will have to search for a double chin or lines on your neck. Girls and women who wear flats have a better chance for a double chin and lines on their neck than women who wear high heels.

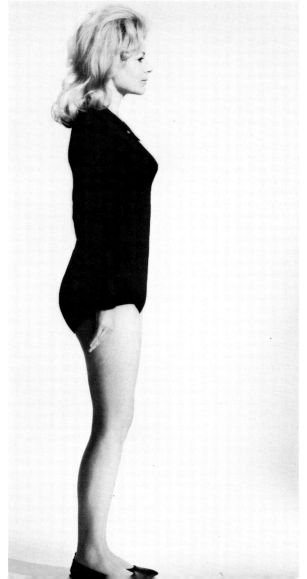

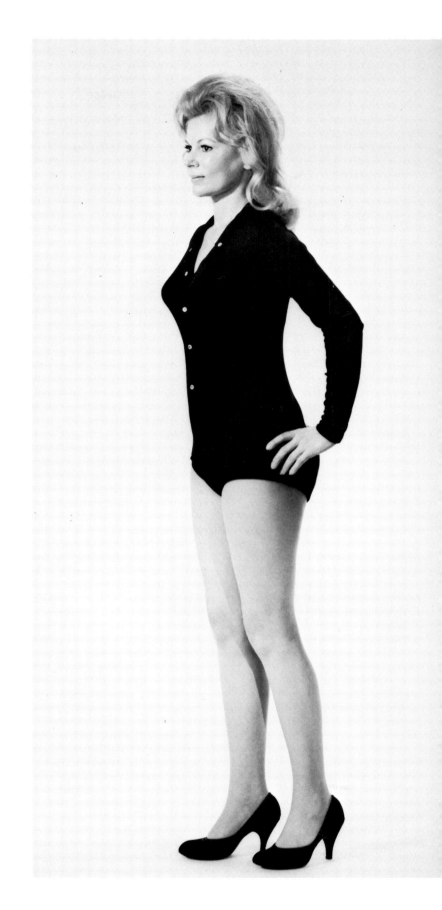

WALKING: Now try walking in the same position you have just learned for standing — body and head upright, chin forward and level, shoulder blades back and down, and the weight of your body on the balls of your feet, especially on the joints of your big toes. If the mirror test shows that even though you sit, stand and walk in the right position, there is still a sign of a double chin (which is caused by collapsed muscles), start with the corrective exercise for double chin.

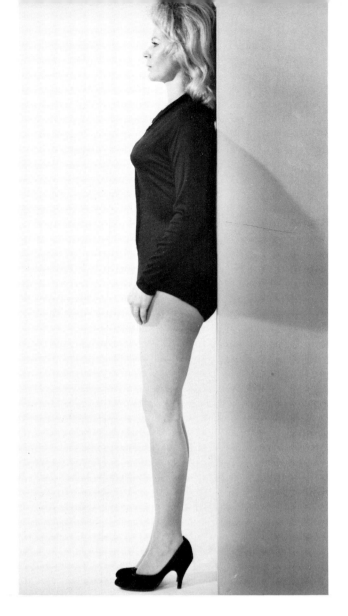

EXERCISE FOR POSTURE COR-RECTION: While standing, check your posture in front of a full-length mirror. Stand with your back against a wall, feet together, but about 2-3 inches away from the wall. Keep shoulder blades straight against the wall and pull them somewhat down. See that the chin is level. Now straighten out the hollowness at your back by flattening it against the wall. First pull the abdominal muscles and then the buttock muscles in and hold this position.

EXCERCISE TO PREVENT A DOUBLE CHIN: caused by flaccid neck muscles. Daily roll your head, bending it backward and forward; then turn it to the left and the right three times in succession. Furthermore, when someone calls you from behind, do not turn your entire body around as if your head were welded to your body, but turn your head alone, as a young girl would do.

DOUBLE CHIN CONTAINING FATTY DEPOSITS: cannot be removed by exercises but only through dieting and/or plastic surgery.

DOWAGER HUMP: Do this before getting up in the morning. Move shoulders to edge of bed. Slowly drop head backward, then raise and return to starting position. Be sure you keep shoulders and feet flat on bed and that only the head moves. Also exercise No. 2 for Jowls will help you to get rid of a dowager hump.

CREPE — LIKE — NECK SKIN: Can be treated very successfully with Senta Maria Runge's "TEARS OF VENUS" neck oil.

*Are you by chance
a slouching secretary??*

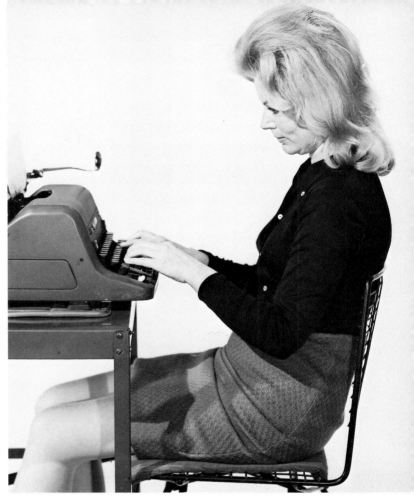

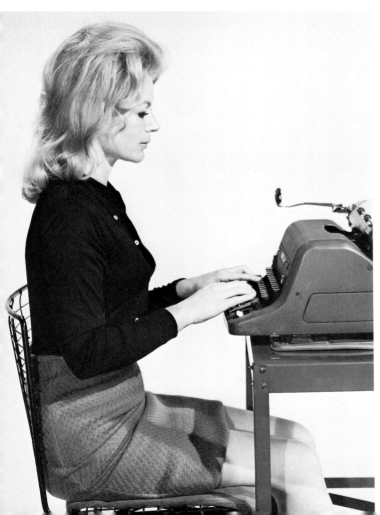

or a graceful one??

Jowls.

When you study the muscle face on page 80 you will notice a jowl is an elongation of the upper cheek muscles which have lost the strength of holding themselves firm and up. The consequent "too much" has collected at the bottom in the form of little bags called jowls.

ENCOURAGEMENT:. . . *One morning I went through all of your exercises while my husband was watching. He expressed great amazement when my jowls practically disappeared right before his eyes.*

H. N. J., Sherman Oaks, Calif.

PRELIMINARY PRACTICE:
to isolate and to gain awareness of your jowl muscles

--- May be done in a sitting or standing position. Look into mirror.

--- Apply a thick layer of Senta Maria Runge's Exercise Creme around your eyes where lines may appear when you squint.

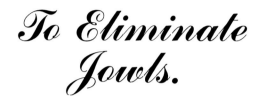

To Eliminate Jowls.

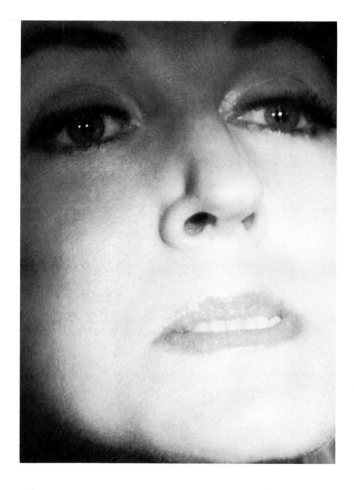

a) Bring lower teeth and jaw forward.

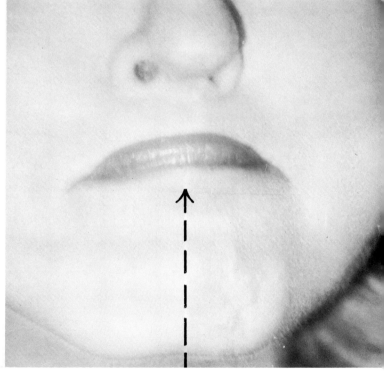

b) Pull over upper teeth and lip as far as possible. Grip top lip firmly with your bottom teeth.

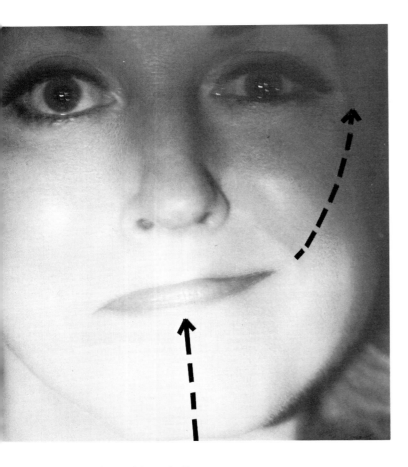
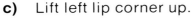

c) Lift left lip corner up.

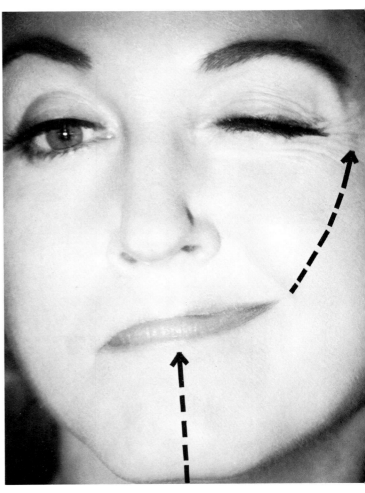

d) While holding the above position squint left eye.

e) Consciously and gradually release squint; return lip corner and mouth to normal position.

Practice the same on the right side of your face, lifting right lip corner and squinting right eye.

Purpose: Learn to lift up the lip corners freely.

Note: This is possible only when the face and particularly the lip corners are kept relaxed since tension hinders muscles from moving. Some people can do it instantly, others have to practice for some time until they can do it.

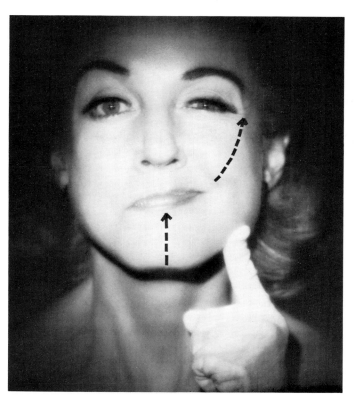

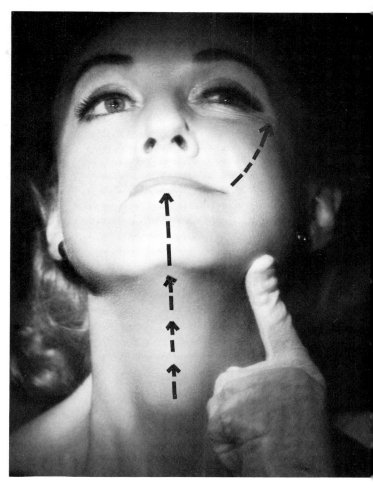

--- Apply a thick layer of Senta Maria Runge's Exercise Cremé around your eyes where lines may appear when you squint.

--- Apply several drops of Senta Maria Runge's Vita-Ex throat oil on the skin of your front neck.

Hold mirror in hand.

Step 1. Sit on edge of chair, torso and head upright, chin level.

Step 2. Touch the center of left jowl with point of left forefinger and apply steps a-d of PRELIMI-NARY PRACTICE.

Step 3. In this position and while keeping shoulders straight and immobile jut chin straight forward, then pull chin up until head rests in back. (Check with mirror to see that teeth, lip corner and squint have not slipped.)

Step 4. Try to feel a good pull on left jowl, at the point where the finger touches.

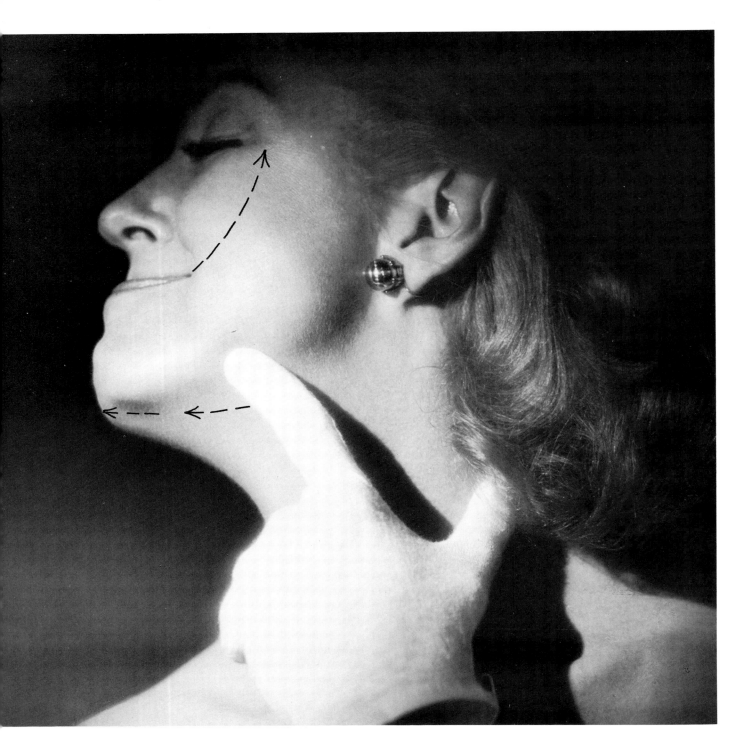

Step 5. While keeping this pull steady, turn head to right, gradually in an even line until you can look over your right shoulder.

Step 6. Still maintaining the pull in the correct spot, turn head to the front, gradually and in an even line.

Step 7. Return head, mouth corner, lip and eye muscles.

Repeat two more times on left jowl, then apply exercise three times on right jowl, turning to your left shoulder.

Purpose: Expanding designated muscles by moving the head in opposite direction.

Note: A good pull at the center of the jowl muscles is necessary throughout the turning of the head. A good pull can be felt by
   ··· keeping the head far enough back when turning
   ··· keeping lip corner up high enough
   keeping eye tightly shut
   ··· breathing normally.

If the pull in the jowl has been lost during the action, then one of the above mentioned instructions has not been followed.

Refer: Page (58) - AIM: 15 steps; return head in 10 steps.

Frequency: Once a day on each side three times in succession.

Results: Immediate when 10-step-movements have been applied correctly.

Back Of Cheeks And Temples.

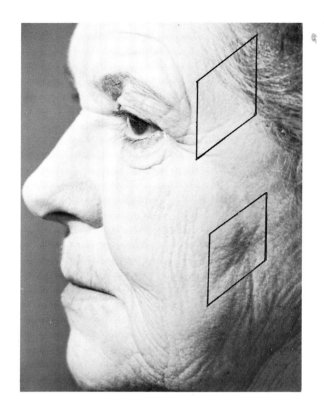

The facial area at the temples and behind the cheeks may sink in due to atrophying muscles in this area, particularly when the muscles involved become inactive due to the removal of some back teeth.

ENCOURAGEMENT: . . . *I am so thrilled and grateful that I was able to round out my face with your exercises.*

B. L., Beverly Hills, Calif.

To Firm & Fill Out Sunken= In Temples & Back Of Cheeks.

Thus bestowing a more youthful roundness to the face.

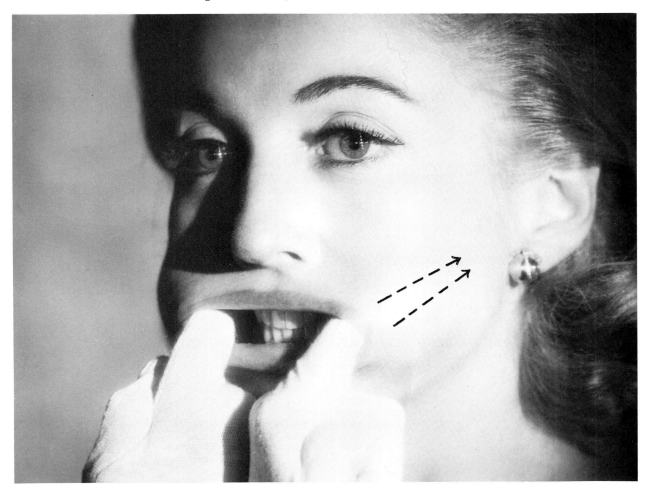

- - - Sitting or standing position. Look into mirror.

Step 1. Keep the bite closed.

Step 2. Insert index fingers in mouth and slide them along the teeth, backward until the fingers have reached the end. There you will realize that each index finger is between the teeth and a strong muscle wall.

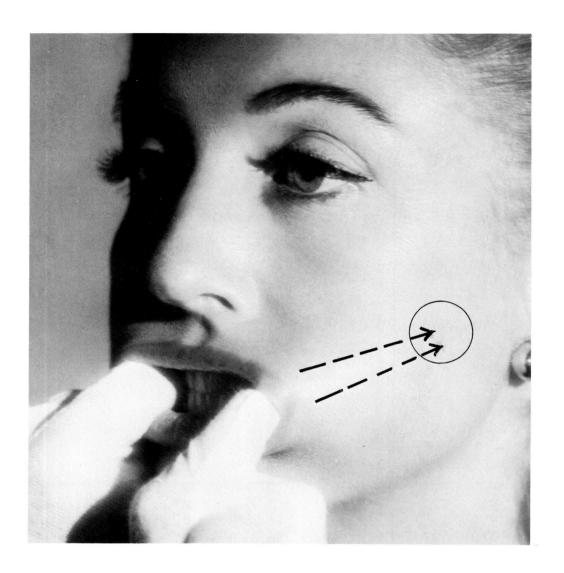

Step 3. Push the muscle wall outward with the index finger tip and very firmly hold this position for resistance.

Step 4. By simply trying to bite the back teeth together from soft to hard, you will feel tremendous pressure against the resistance (in this case your finger tips) which must be held firmly throughout the exercise. Increase the pressure for at least five counts and release pressure in the same slow fashion.

Step 5. Release resistance.

Purpose: Expanding designated muscles through added pressure against resistance.

Note: Pressure must be kept equal on both sides of the face to assure a balanced even appearance. If you prefer, an adequate article of soft but firm material may be substituted for the index fingers. Do not exercise with long finger nails, as the membrane inside the mouth is delicate and long nails could injure the gum.

Refer: Page (58) - AIM: 10 steps: return muscles in 10 steps.

Frequency: Once a day three times in succession.

Results: In some faces instantly: in others after a few days. (Also apply Exercise No. 3-A)

ISOMETRIC EXERCISE

To Firm & Fill Out Sunken-In Temples & Back Of Cheeks.

(Use in alternation with or addition to Exercise No. 3)

- - - Sitting or standing position.

Step 1. Place a thick cloth between teeth and fingers and pull the jaw down.

Step 2. Hold the jaw firmly down while at the same time trying
a) to close the mouth
b) to laugh in back of cheeks.

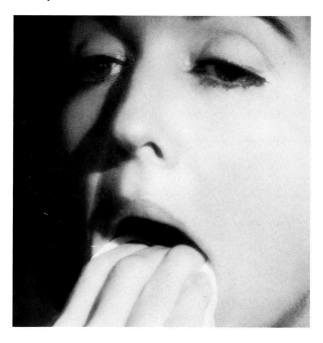

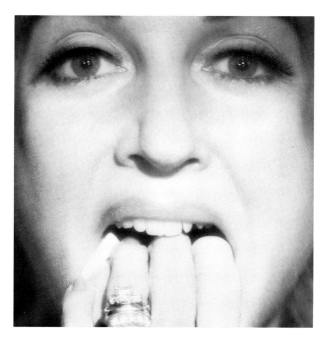

Purpose: To contract muscles through added pressure against resistance.

Note: Work gently and gradually. so as not to dislocate your jaw.

Refer: Page (58) - AIM: 15 counts: relax in 10 counts.

Frequency: 5 times in succession.

Results: After a few days.

Lower Cheeks.

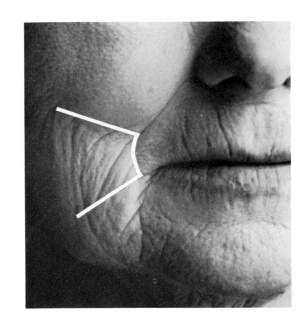

Loss of tone and consequent elongation of the muscles constituting our lower cheeks may result in flabbiness, hollowness, and vertical lines in the lower cheeks. A once cute looking dimple will unavoidably turn into a vertical line through elongation of its muscles unless it is kept firm through this exercise.

ENCOURAGEMENT: . . . *I am in the early stages of exercising my lower cheeks and the results have been marvelous!!!*

G. R., Long Beach, Calif.

For Firming
Lower Cheeks & Mouth-Corners

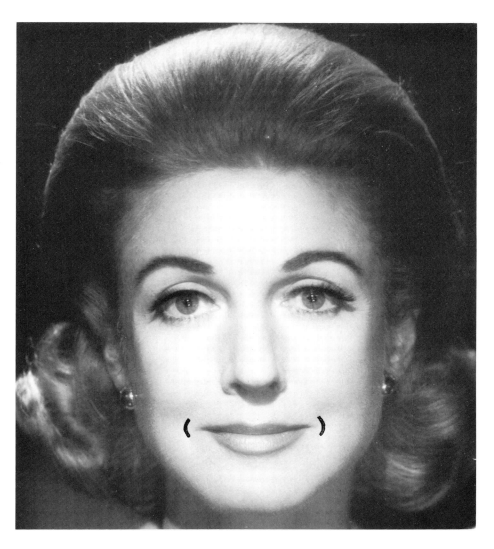

Observe the muscle face on page 80. Notice that the smile line is the point of action of our smiling muscles which perform horizontally back to the ears and constitute the larger part of our lower cheeks.

- - - Sit, stand or lie down. Look into mirror.

- - - With eyebrow pencil emphasize smile line (as in photo) on each side of face. A smile line is the curved line approximately ¼ inch in back of the lip corner. Some people have to smile to see their smile lines. These smiling muscles attach at their front end (point of action) to the skin, thus forming the smile line.

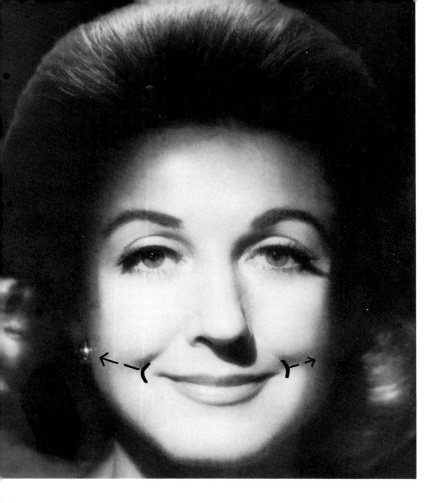

- - - Practice on both sides of face simultaneously.

a) Teeth and lips stay together. however they must be relaxed and limp.

b) Through the action of "smiling back" move your smile lines horizontally back toward the earlobes as indicated by arrows. Range of this muscle movement is approximately ¾ to one inch. consequently you have to see your smile lines moving back such a distance.

c) Return smile lines consciously to starting position.

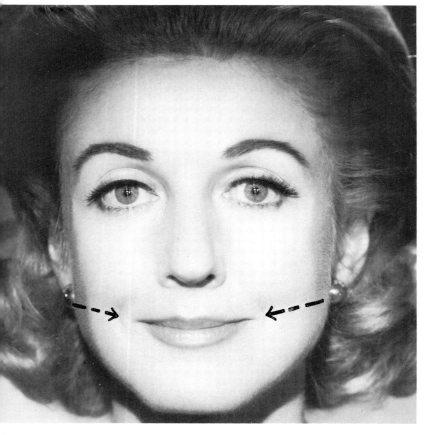

Purpose: Moving designated muscles freely and in their fullest range without tension of lips or help of other surrounding muscles.

Note: When lines appear around your eyes while smiling back. you have used the wrong muscles. No skin around your eyes must move when you smile "back."

Refer: Page (58) - AIM: 10 steps: return muscles in 10 steps.

Frequency: Once a day 3 times in succession until you have conquered the AIM.

- - - Do not attempt unless you have mastered the PRELIMINARY PRACTICE.

- - - Sitting position preferred. Look into mirror.

- - - Wear cosmetic gloves to avoid slipping.

Step 1. Place one or two finger points directly under each smile line which we have identified as the point of action.

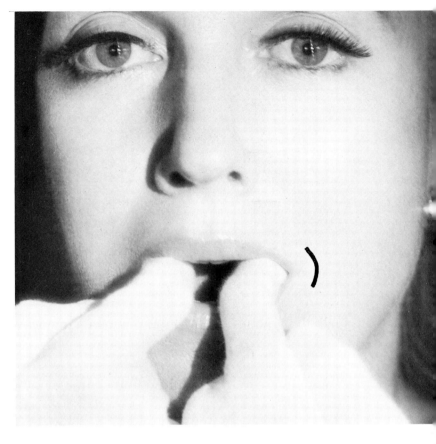

Step 2. Push smile lines somewhat out with your finger points.

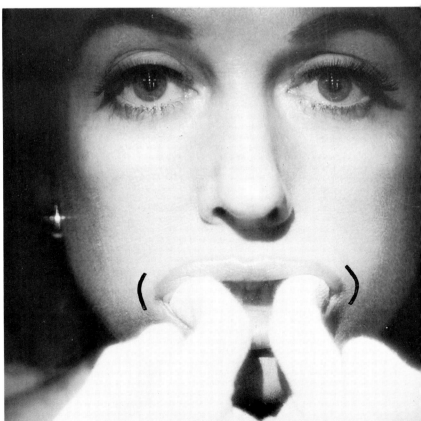

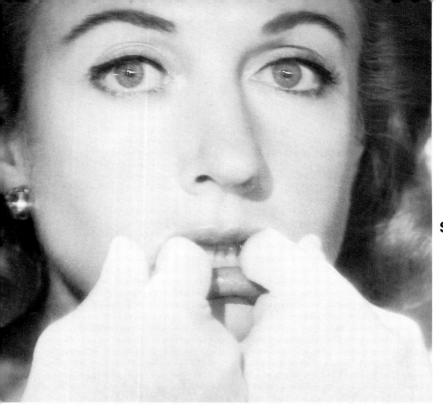

Step 3. Grip smile lines as with a pair of pliers firmly with thumbs outside and finger points inside the mouth. You are now holding the smiling muscles at their front end (point of action). Make absolutely sure you are holding the smile line (end of lower cheek muscles) and not a little in front which would cause the lower cheek muscles to stretch.

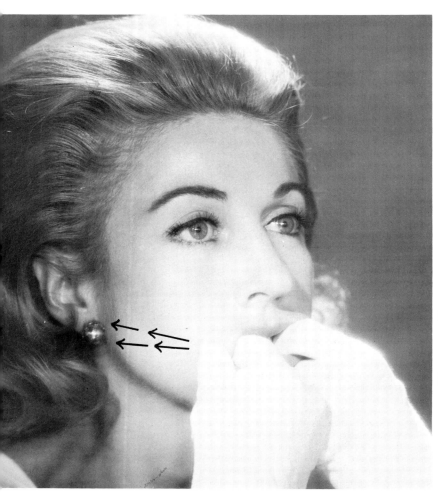

Step 4. Pull gripped smile lines forward and hold this position for resistance.

Step 5. Smile as you have learned in the PRELIMINARY PRACTICE by trying to move your smile line against finger resistance which, of course, causes your smiling muscles to expand. Think of a rubberband which you hold and expand.

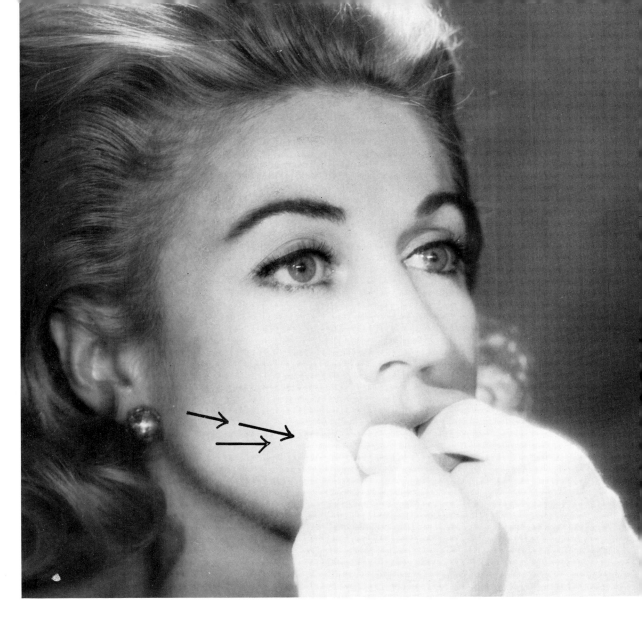

Step 6. Consciously return muscles involved to starting position.

Step 7. Remove finger resistance.

Purpose: Expanding designated muscles to their fullest capacity which is approximately ¾ to one inch.

Note: Your resistance must never move during the entire exercise. Watch that your smiling lines do not slip out of your grip. Should one hand be too weak to maintain firm resistance, you may work on one smiling line at a time by holding resistance with both hands.

Refer: Page (58) - AIM: 15 steps: return muscles in 10 steps.

Frequency: Once a day three times in succession. Hands must be removed and results observed after each performance.

Results: A correct performance with more than three-step-movements will show immediate results.

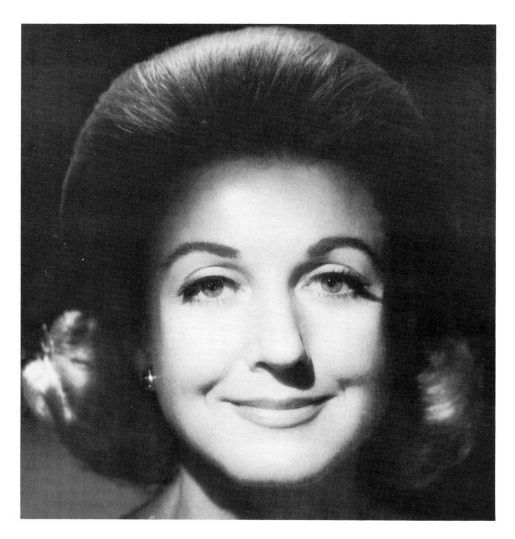

ADDITIONAL SUGGESTIONS TO "SMILING BACK"

A natural youthful smile is always accomplished by the "smile lines". However, with increasing birthdays people have the tendency to smile by "pushing" with their lip corners either back or down. This habit, in time, will cause the smile lines to disappear and instead create a distracting looking pouch-line from the lip corners down.

In such cases, in order to be able to learn my smiling exercise, one has to re-establish the natural youthful smile by keeping lip corners relaxed and concentrating solely on smiling with the smile lines. To re-train those muscles may take some time and patience as does every change of habit. It is very worthwhile working to establish your youthful smile for your daily wear.

Do you freeze while looking into your mirror? Then practice at first without looking into the mirror. Think of something that may trigger your natural smile, hold it in this position and look at your mirrored image. Now return your smile lines controlled while you count. This is an excellent way of acquainting yourself with your smile line muscles and to bring them under control.

For Building Up Muscle Flesh In Lower Cheeks & Firming Mouth Corners.

Step 1. Place entire index finger inside mouth corners sliding them horizontally back, as far as fingers will go.

Step 2. Set resistance by pushing muscle flesh outward with fingers and hold fingers firm in this position.

Step 3. Push muscles against finger resistance gradually from soft to hard for 10-15 counts.

Step 4. Release muscles gradually in 10 counts to starting position.

Frequency: Once a day 3-4 times in succession.

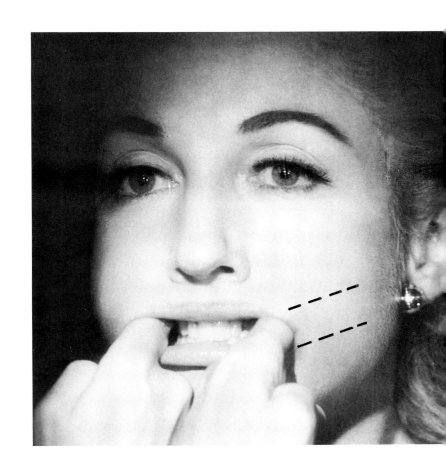

Pouches.

The muscle face on page (80) will reveal to you that the pouches beside the chin are an accumulation of elongated upper cheek muscles, in particular the Zygomaticus. (A small percentage of the pouch may also be contributed by the lower cheek muscles.) Removing the pouches will lift your face greatly and consequently will remove many years from your facial appearance.

ENCOURAGEMENT: . . . *and I am very pleased with the results, as my pouches and jowl bags have vanished completely.*

Mrs. A. C., Gardena, Calif.

PRELIMINARY PRACTICE:
(to isolate and to gain awareness of the muscles causing the pouches)

To Eliminate Pouches.

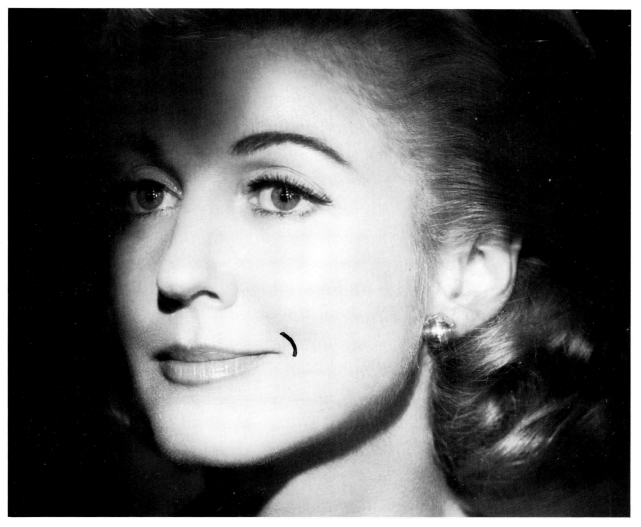

--- Sitting or standing position; mirror in front.

--- Apply thick layer of Senta Maria Runge's Exercise Creme around your eyes where lines may appear when doing this exercise.

a) With eyebrow pencil emphasize smile line on each side of face. A smile line is the curved line approximately ¼ inch in back of the lip corner. Some people have to smile to see their smile lines.

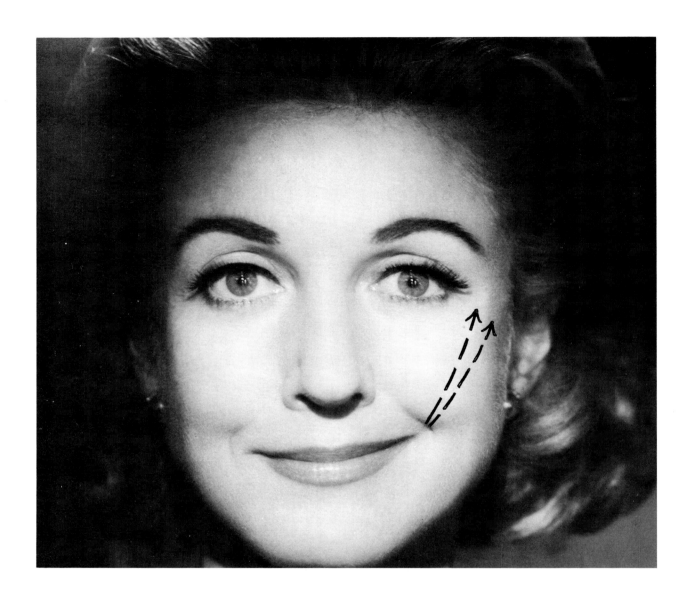

b) Hold teeth and lips together, however keep them relaxed and limp.

c) Practice lifting smile line (on one side at a time) diagonally upward in the direction indicated by arrows.

d) Consciously and gradually return smile line to normal.

Purpose; To move designated muscles freely and in their fullest range, approximately ¾ to one inch without tension or help by surrounding muscles.

Refer: Page (58) - AIM: 7-8 steps; return in 7-8 steps.

Note: If a pouch is not corrected in time, it will cause jowls, as an extended droopiness. This particular exercise will also remedy sagging mouth corners.

Frequency: As often as you may wish until the AIM has been accomplished.

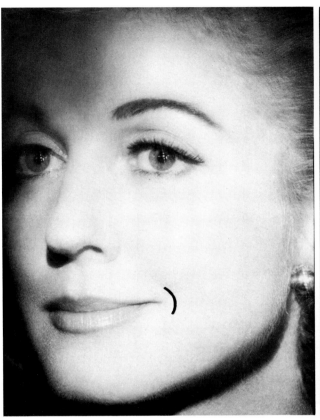 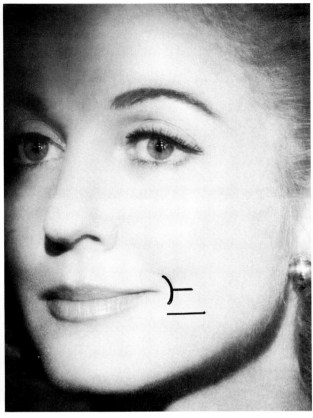

- - - Do not attempt unless you have mastered the PRELIMINARY PRACTICE.

- - - Apply thick layer of Senta Maria Runge's Exercise Cremé around your eyes where lines may appear when doing this exercise.

- - - Sitting position with elbows resting on table. Look into mirror.

- - - Wear cosmetic gloves to avoid slipping.

a) With eyebrow pencil emphasize your smile lines as in the PRELIMINARY PRACTICE.

b) Draw two horizontal lines, the first line starting at the center of the smile lines and the second one about ½ inch apart.

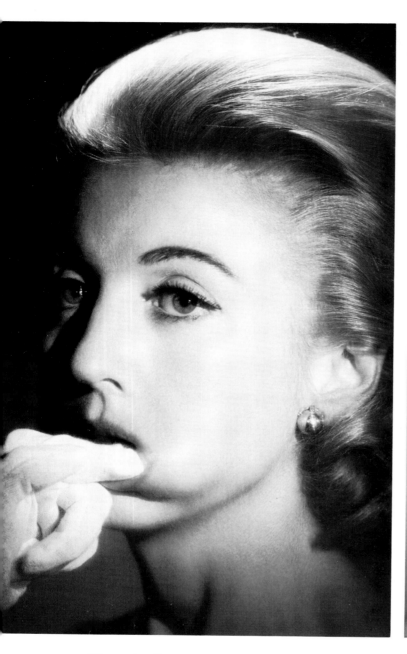 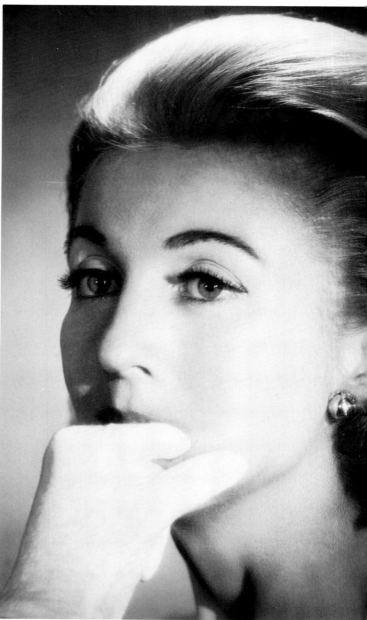

Step 1. On one side at a time insert index finger into mouth, pushing out flatly (not pointed) the area between the lines.

Step 2. Now grip the designated muscle area (between the two lines) as with a pair of pliers firmly between thumb outside and finger inside the mouth.

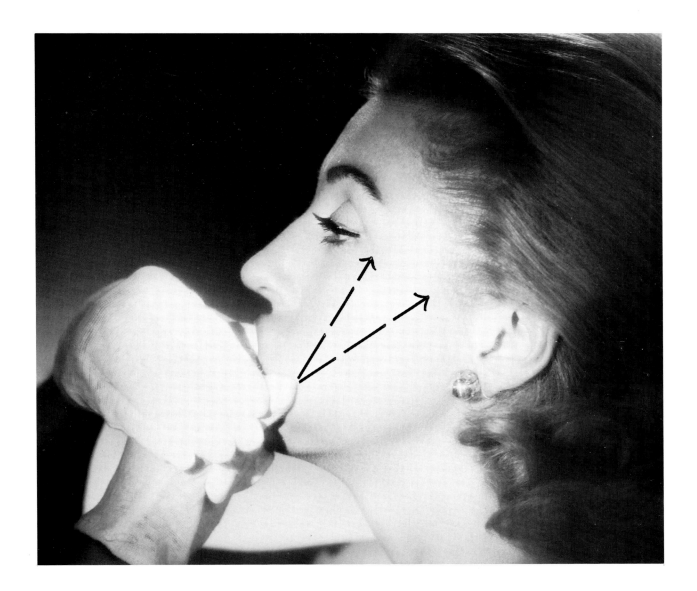

Step 3. Support the grip with the other hand.

Step 4. Hold this position firm as a resistance while trying to lift the smile line as you have learned in the PRELIMINARY PRACTICE.

Step 5. Consciously and gradually return muscles to starting position.

Step 6. Release finger resistance.

Purpose: Expanding designated muscles in their fullest range.

Note: Your resistance must never move during the entire exercise. Watch that your muscles do not slip out of your grip.

Refer: Page (58) - AIM: 15 steps; return in 10 steps.

Frequency: Once a day 3 times in succession on each side of the face. Hands must be removed and results observed after each performance.

Results: A correct performance with more than 3-step-movements will show immediate results.

Upper Cheeks

The law of gravity is that things fall downward from top to bottom. The upper cheek muscle flesh shifts downward, leaving hollowness beneath the eye-circle and below the cheek bones. As the weight shifts down it collects at the laugh line and at the lower face, causing furrows, pouches, and jowls.

The collapse of the upper cheek muscles alone may cause more than fifty percent of the aging in a face and consequently the elimination of the same may contribute equally to a younger look.

ENCOURAGEMENT: . . . *I have lifted my sagging countenance and friends just stare at me. I just celebrated my 62nd birthday and most people take me for 42, thanks to you.*

B. C., Ventura, Calif.

For Lifting & Firming Upper Cheeks & Removing The Furrows Of Laugh Lines.

Observe the muscle face on page (80). Notice that the upper cheeks consist largely of four muscle sections called Quadratus, Labii, Superioris and Zygomaticus which run from the temples and eye-ring-muscles toward the nose-mouth line. The upper cheek muscles attach at their point of action to the skin, thus forming the line from the nose to the mouth which we use for laughing or smiling up. For the exercises let us call the muscle-line extending from nose to mouth the "laugh line" and where this line curves we shall call it "smile line."

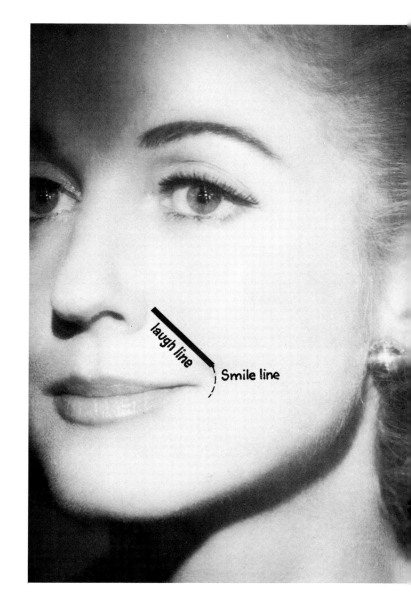

laugh line

Smile line

PRELIMINARY PRACTICE:
(to isolate and to gain awareness of your upper cheek muscles)

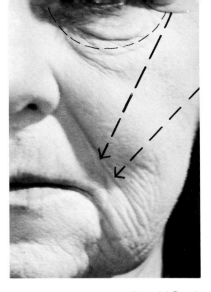

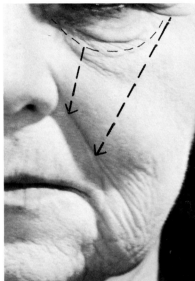

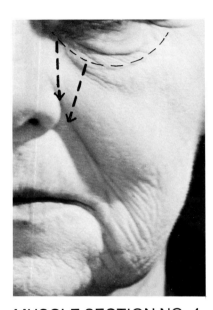

MUSCLE SECTION NO. 4, when collapsed, causes an overlap on the laugh line next to the nose and consequently hollowness below the eye-circle next to the nose.

MUSCLE SECTION No. 3, when collapsed, causes hollowness beneath the eye-circle and an overlap in its location on the laugh line.

MUSCLE SECTION NO. 1 & 2, when losing their battle against gravity's pull, show a devastating "landslide" due to their large size and area. The Muscle Face on page 80 will explain why loss of tone and consequent elongation of these muscles cause

a) hollowness at their point of origin (below the cheek bone)
b) flabbiness and overlap on their location on the laugh line
c) droopy mouth corners
d) pouches beside chin
e) jowl bags

In cases where all four Upper Cheek Muscle Groups have collapsed — indicated by an even, continuous overlap on the laugh line — I recommend the "General Upper Cheek Exercise." If only Muscle Sections 3 & 4 show signs of relaxation, and none are shown by 1 & 2, work specifically with 3 & 4. It is Muscle Section 1 & 2 however, which most likely will show elongation before the two smaller Upper Cheek Muscles of 3 & 4 do. In such instance it is best to work exclusively with Muscle Section 1 & 2 as instructed on pages 132 & 133, without permitting Muscle Section 3 & 4 to move. If all four Upper Cheek Muscles require attention, but particularly Muscle Section 1 & 2, then it may be desirable to perform the Isometric as shown on pages 132 & 133, in addition to the General Upper Cheek Exercise.

--- Sitting position. Look into mirror.

--- Apply thick layer of Senta Maria Runge's Exercise Cremé around your eyes.

a) With eyebrow pencil emphasize line from nose to mouth (laugh line) which is the point of action for the Upper Cheek muscles.

b) Mark your upper cheeks in four sections.

MUSCLE SECTION NO. 1: Mark with a line starting at the smile/laugh line and running diagonally toward the temple.

MUSCLE SECTION NO. 2: Mark with a line that points diagonally toward the ending of the brows.

MUSCLE SECTION NO. 3: Start the line at the center of your laugh line, ending at the center of the circle underneath the eyes.

MUSCLE SECTION NO. 4: Start on the laugh line next to the nostril and end at the eye-circle beginning next to the nose.

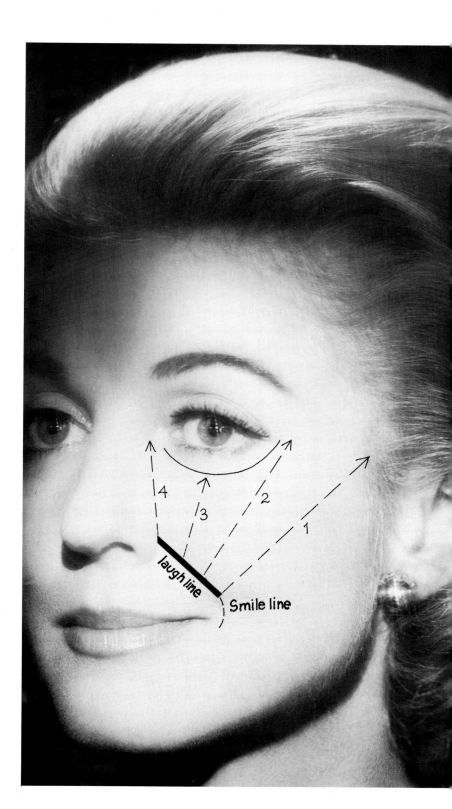

- - - Practice on both cheeks simultaneously and/or each cheek individually.

c) Teeth together and lip loose and relaxed.

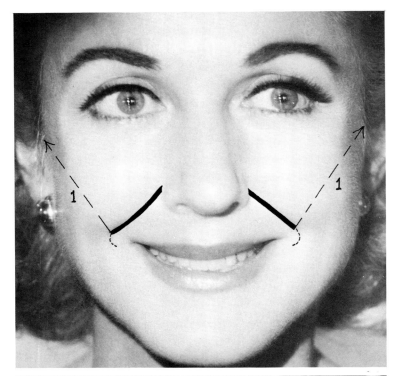

Move No. 1 Muscle Section by lifting smile line in the direction of arrow No. 1

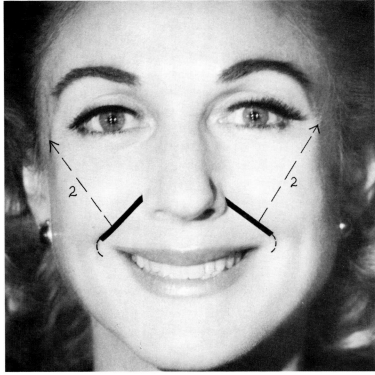

Move No. 2 Muscle Section by lifting laugh line in the direction of arrow No. 2

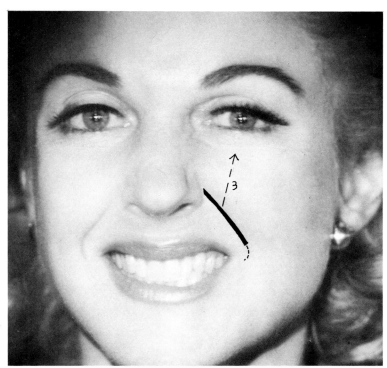

Move No. 3 Muscle Section by lifting laugh line in the direction of arrow No. 3

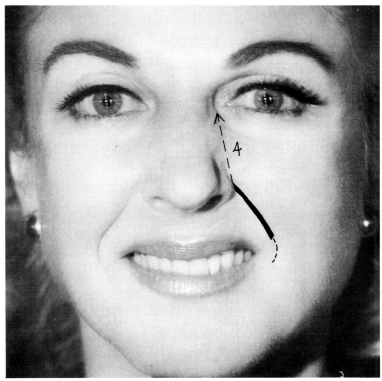

Move No. 4 Muscle section by lifting laugh line in the direction of arrow No. 4

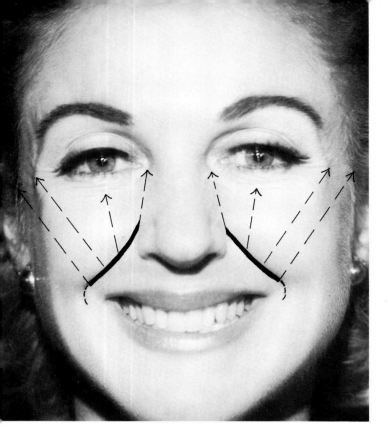

d) Now practice moving all four muscle groups together (which is your entire upper cheek).

e) Return upper cheek muscles consciously to starting position.

Purpose: Moving designated muscles freely and in their fullest range without tension of lips or help of other surrounding muscles.

Note: The range of movement for muscle section No. 1 and No. 2 is approximately one inch, consequently, you have to see your laugh line moving such a distance. The action is your natural "smiling upward."

The range of movement for muscle sections No. 3 and No. 4 is approximately ½ inch. The action is a "sneer."

Since the four upper cheek muscle groups attach at their bottom to the lip muscles and at their top to the eye-ring-muscles, watch that you do not relieve the cheek muscles of their work by pushing them from the bottom with your lip, or by pulling from the top with the eye-ring-muscles (through squinting).

The point of action is in your laugh line. Further note, that if your smile line moves backward horizontally instead of diagonally toward the temples, you have moved the lower cheek muscles (which perform horizontally back toward the ear-lobes) instead of the upper cheek muscles.

Refer: Page (58). - AIM: 10 steps; return muscles in 10 steps.

Frequency: Once a day 3 times in succession until you have conquered your AIM.

GENERAL ISOMETRIC EXERCISE FOR LIFTING UPPER CHEEKS:

- - - Do not attempt unless you have mastered the PRELIMINARY PRACTICE.

- - - Apply thick layer of Senta Maria Runge's Exercise Creme around eye area.

- - - Sitting position, with elbows resting on table. Look into mirror.

- - - Wear cosmetic gloves to avoid slipping.

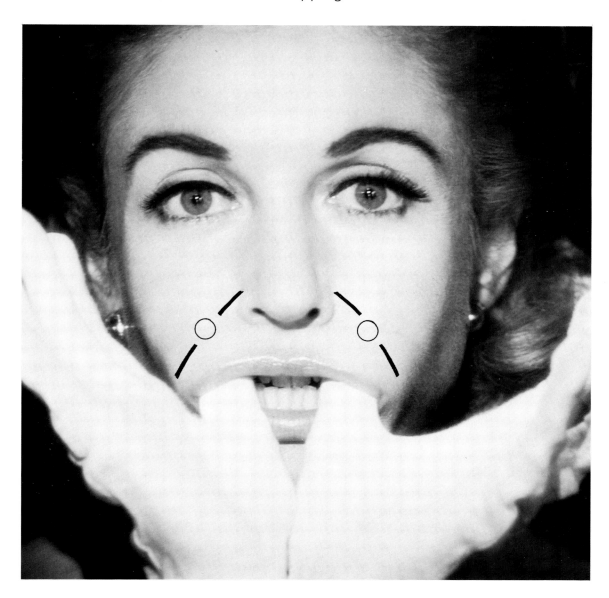

Step 1. Place point of thumbs inside mouth directly under laugh line (muscle) about the center of the laugh line between muscles indicated as No.'s 2 and 3.

Step 2. Push laugh line (muscle) somewhat out.

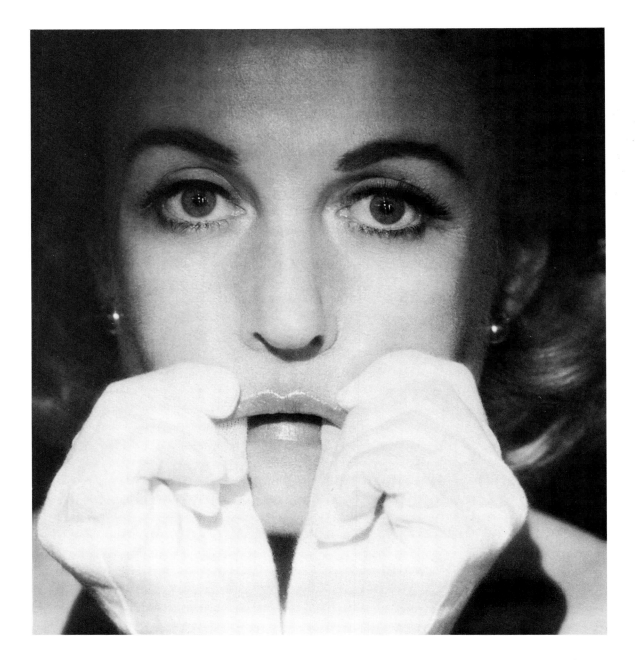

Step 3. Grip the <u>laugh line</u> as with a pair of pliers firmly with thumb inside and the bony part of the first joint of the index finger outside your mouth. You are now holding the upper cheek muscles at their point of action. Make absolutely sure you are holding the laugh line muscle and not a little below which would cause the upper cheek muscles to stretch.

Step 4. Pull gripped laugh line somewhat down.

Step 5. Hold this position as a firm resistance.

Step 6. Smile with all four muscle sections (upper cheek generally) gradually as you have learned in the PRELIMINARY PRACTICE. Think of a rubber band which you hold and expand.

Step 7. Consciously return muscles involved to starting position.

Step 8. Remove finger resistance.

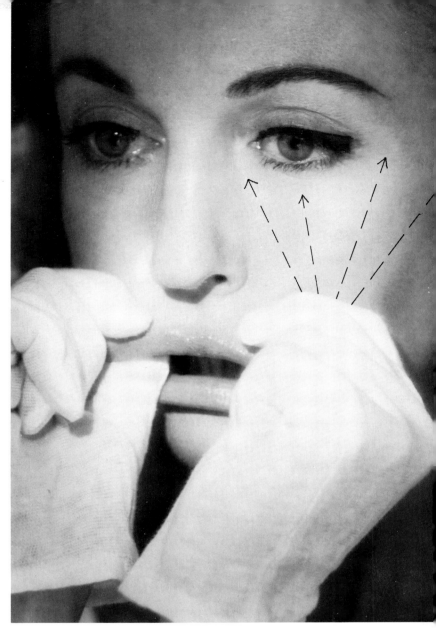

Purpose: Expanding designated muscles within their fullest range.

Note: Consider everything said under ''NOTE'' in the PRELIMINARY PRACTICE. - - - Your resistance must never move during the entire exercise. Watch that your laugh line does not slip out of the grip.

Refer: Page (58). - AIM: 15 steps; return muscles in 10 steps.

Frequency: Once a day 3 times in succession. Hands must be removed and results observed after each performance.

Results: A correct performance with more than 3-step-movements will show an immediate lift, a firming and filling out of the cheeks and lessening in the overlap at the laugh line.

ISOMETRIC EXERCISE

- - - Do not attempt unless you have mastered the PRELIMINARY PRACTICE.

- - - Apply thick layer of Senta Maria Runge's Exercise Cremé around eye area.

- - - Sitting position, with elbows resting on table. Look into mirror.

- - - Wear cosmetic gloves to avoid slipping.

WHEN CORRECTING MUSCLE SECTION NO. 1 & 2

Step 1. Place point of thumb inside mouth directly under laugh line at the point of action of muscle section No. 1 & 2.

Step 2. Push laugh line (muscle) at this point somewhat out.

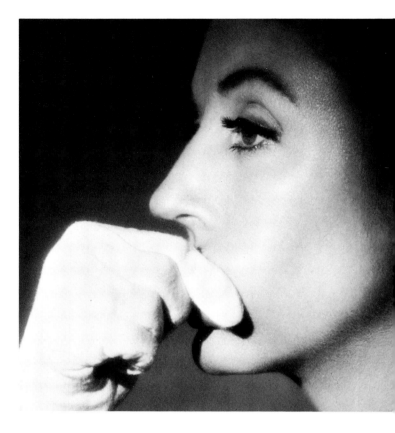

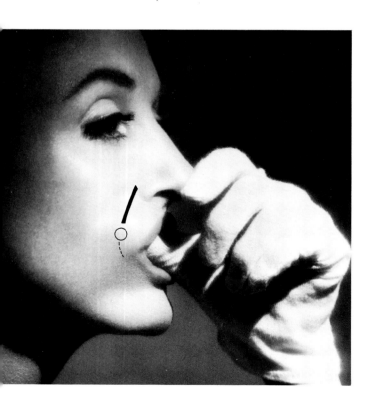

Step 3. Grip the laugh line (muscle) at this point as with a pair of pliers firmly with the thumb inside and the bony part of the first joint of the index finger outside the mouth. You are now holding muscle section No. 1 & 2 at their end (point of action). Make absolutely sure you are holding the laugh line muscle and not a little below.

Step 4. Pull gripped muscles somewhat down.

Step 5. Hold this position as a firm resistance.

Step 6. Smile muscle section No. 1 & 2 in their direction as you have learned in the PRELIMINARY PRACTICE. Think of a rubber band which you hold and expand.

Step 7. Consciously return muscles involved to starting position.

Step 8. Remove finger resistance.

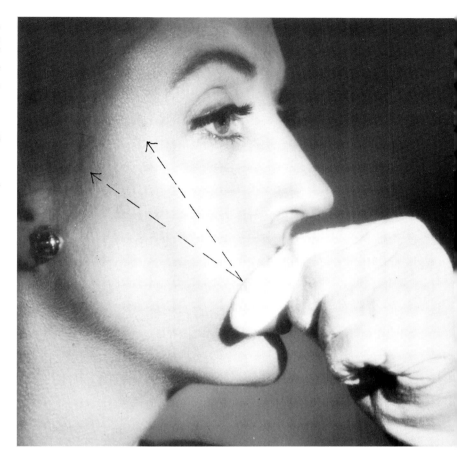

Purpose: Expanding designated muscle section within its fullest range, which is about one inch.

Note: Your resistance must never move during the entire exercise. Watch that your muscle grip does not escape through slipping. You may exercise both sides together or one side at a time, holding the resistance as shown above.

Refer: Page (58). - AIM: 15 steps for muscle sections No. 1 and No. 2

Frequency: Once a day 3 times in succession. Resistance must be removed and results observed after each performance.

Results: A correct performance with more than 3 steps will show immediate results by lifting and firming the cheek in the exercised area.

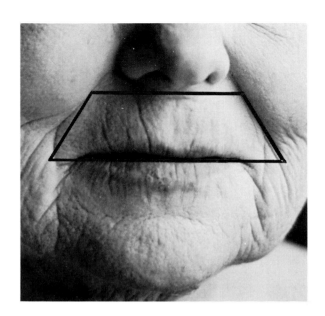

Upper Lip.

The muscle structure of a lip does not reveal its loss of tone and consequent collapse through elongation as do most other facial muscles. Lack of circulation in this area causes muscular atrophy (disappearance), hence the lips become thinner and thinner as time goes on. The lip loses its contour and wrinkles form. Only a full lip is a Youth-Full lip.

ENCOURAGEMENT: . . . *my lips are taking on fullness and shape once more. God bless you for revealing to us your method.*

M. S. S., Beverly Hills, Calif.

To Restore Fullness & Contour In The Upper Lip.

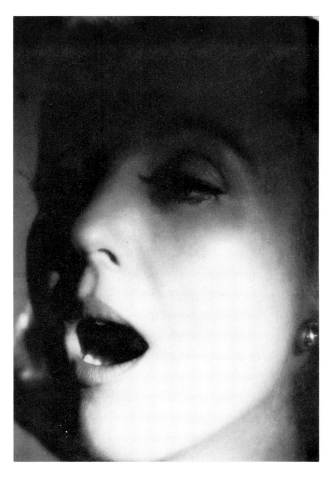

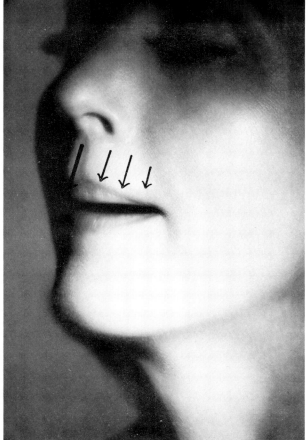

- - - Sitting or standing position. Look into mirror.

Step 1. Pretend to yawn and open mouth with about one and a half inches between the upper and lower front teeth.

Step 2. Keep teeth in this position. While holding upper lip somewhat away from the teeth, move upper lip slowly downward.

Step 3. Consciously return lip gradually to starting position.

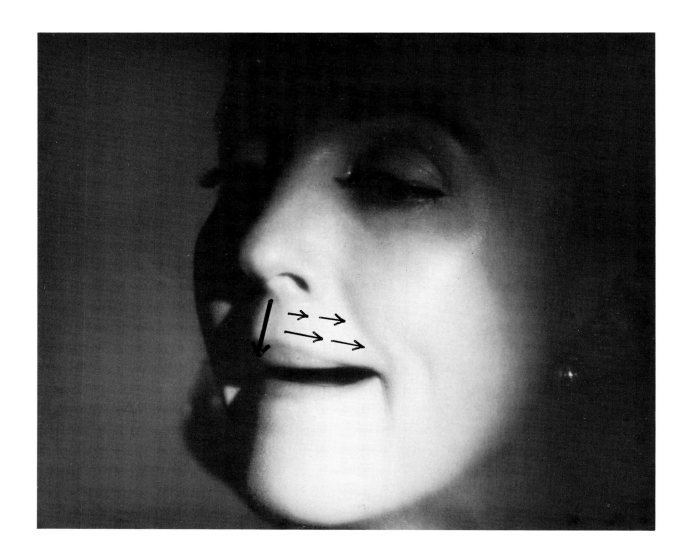

Purpose: Expanding designated muscles freely and in their fullest range, approximately ¼ - ½ inch without tension or help by surrounding muscles.

Note: The middle part of the lip (see longest arrow) must always move ahead of the other lip muscles, thus avoiding the O-form which does form lines into the lip. Mouth corner muscles stay relaxed during action.

Refer: Page (58). - AIM: 10 steps; return muscles in 10 steps. Once you have conquered the downward movements in 10 steps, you may spread the muscles of the upper lip apart - out of the middle; but not by pulling apart with the mouth corners. AIM: 10 steps; return muscles in 10 steps.

Frequency: Once a day 3-5 times in succession.

Results: May be seen if done correctly after approximately one week.

Eliminating Individual Lines In The Upper Lip.

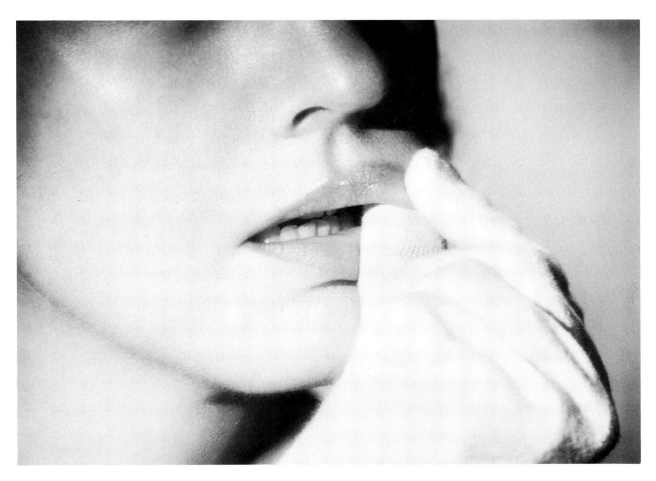

--- Sitting or standing position. Look into mirror.

Step 2. Hold this position as a resistance.

Step 1. Grip bottom end of a lip line between fingers.

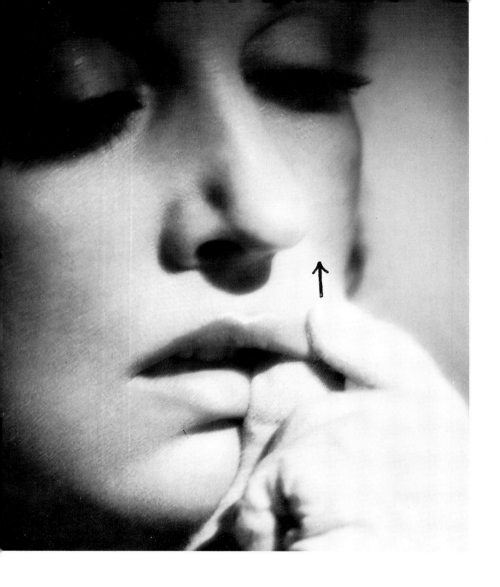

Step 3. Slowly but consciously try to move muscle (line) upward against resistance.

Step 4. Consciously return muscle (line).

Step 5. Release resistance.

Purpose: Expanding designated muscle freely without tension or help by surrounding muscles.

Note: It is important that the muscle movement begins at the resistance, extending toward the laugh line. Make certain you move the muscle (line) and not the muscles next to the line.

Refer: Page (58). - AIM: 10 steps; return muscle in 10 steps.

Frequency: Once a day 3 times in succession.

Results: A correctly performed exercise with more than 5-step-movements will show instant results.

ISOMETRIC EXERCISE:

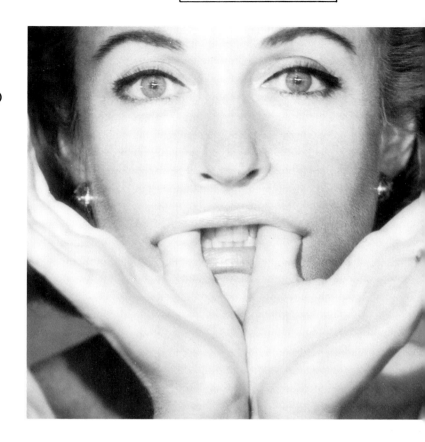

SUBSTITUTE OR ADDITION TO EXERCISE No. 7

The following exercise is very simple, however it is not as effective as Exercise No. 7. It has been designed for those who do not have the patience to learn Exercise No. 7.

- - - Sitting or standing position. Look into mirror.

Step 1. With thumbs push upper lip outward.

Step 2. Hold this position for resistance.

Step 3. Consciously push upper lip muscles against finger resistance by gradually increasing strength of muscle work.

Step 4. Release muscles gradually from their work.

Step 5. Remove finger resistance.

Purpose: Working the muscles against resistance.

Note: Check that you do not cause a line in your face when pushing the muscles against resistance.

Refer: Page (58). - AIM: 10 steps; relax muscles in 10 counts.

Frequency: Once a day 3 times in succession.

Results: May start to show in approximately two weeks if done correctly.

Lower Lip. And Chin.

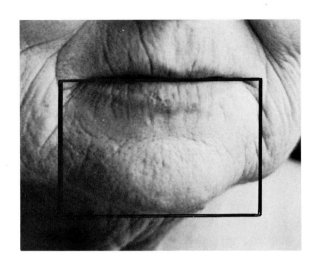

Like the upper lip, the muscle structure of the lower lip and chin reveals its collapse through atrophy (muscle disappearance). Consequently the skin-flesh in this area becomes thinner and the lip and chin take on a shrunken bony appearance as time goes on. The lower lip may fall into wrinkles whereas the skin over the chin bone crepes up. Only a full lip and chin looks Youth-Full!

ENCOURAGEMENT: *. . . Thank you for solving my problem! I have had a crepey and scrawny chin.*

Mrs. R. S., Hollywood, Calif.

To Restore Youth=Full=Ness & Contour To Lower Lip And Chin.

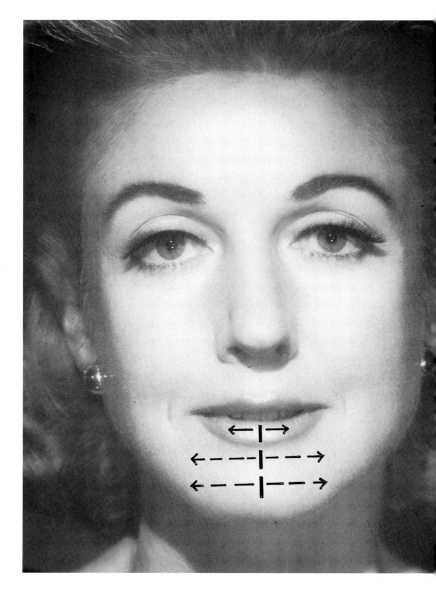

- - - Sitting or standing position. Look into mirror.

Step 1. Teeth closed and lips slightly apart.

Step 2. From the middle of the lower lip and chin move chin-muscle-skin slowly apart.

Step 3. Consciously return lip and chin to starting position.

Purpose: Expanding designated muscles freely and in their fullest range, approximately ¼-½ inch, without tension or help by surrounding muscles.

Note: Watch that the mouth corners do not help by pulling lip and chin apart.

Refer: Page (58). - AIM: 10 steps; return muscles in 10 steps.

Frequency: Once or twice a day 3-5 times in succession.

Results: May be seen if done correctly after approximately one week.

EXERCISE No. 8-A

SUBSTITUTE OR ADDITION TO EXERCISE No. 8

The following exercise is very simple, however, it is not as effective as Exercise No. 8. It has been designed for those who do not have the patience to learn Exercise No. 8.

For Lower Lip

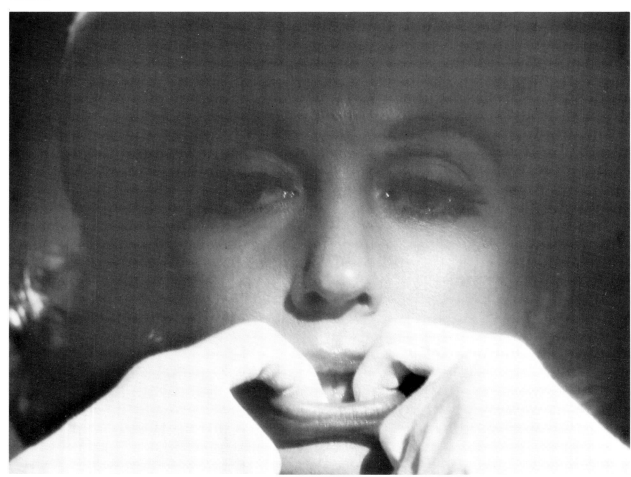

- - - Sitting or standing position. Look into mirror.

Step 1. With index fingers push lower lip outward.

Step 2. Hold this position as a resistance.

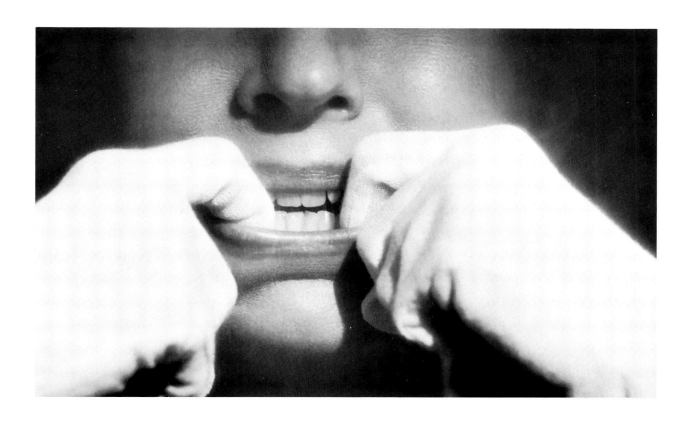

Step 3. Consciously push lower lip (muscles) against finger resistance, gradually increasing muscle work.

Step 4. Release muscles gradually from working.

Step 5. Remove finger resistance.

Purpose: Working the muscles against resistance.

Note: Check that you do not cause a line in the chin area during exercise.

Refer: Page (58). - AIM: 10 steps; return in 10 steps.

Frequency: Once a day 3 times in succession.

Results: May start to show in approximately two weeks if done correctly.

Forehead

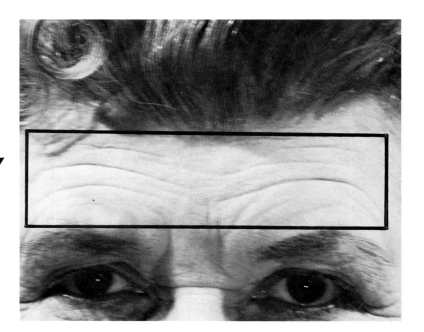

Forehead muscles are expression muscles. Unlike other muscles, expression muscles do not collapse in the form of lines because of inadequate activity. Expression lines are muscles which have formed into lines by the habit of holding them in this position. Horizontal lines on forehead form by the habit of keeping the eyebrows raised.

Since those lines are not an adjunct of aging — young people can have them too — their removal does not add to a younger look, but, indeed, to a more attractive one.

ENCOURAGEMENT: . . . . *I have had wonderful results with my upper face. I removed all of my forehead lines and believe me they were deep.*

Mrs. R. B., Glendale

To Remove Horizontal Lines.

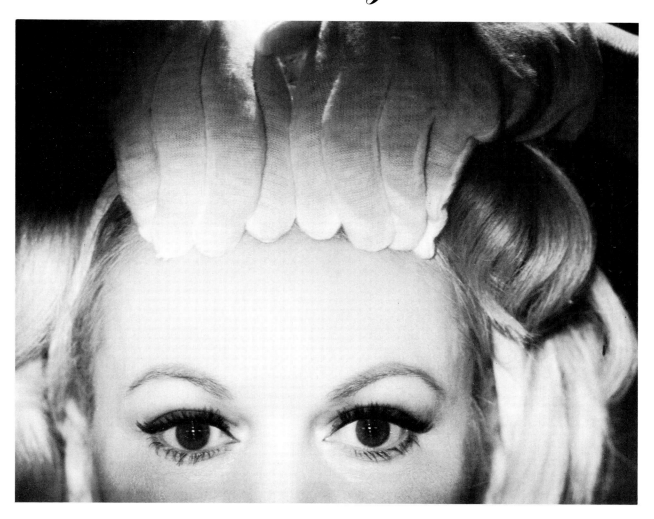

- - - Sitting or standing position. Look into mirror.

- - - Cosmetic gloves may be used to avoid slipping.

Step 1. Place all your fingers - except thumbs - in an even row close above Y O U R topmost horizontal line on forehead.

Step 2. Press fingers tight against the bone.

Step 3. Now with these fingers push the skin upward as much as possible.

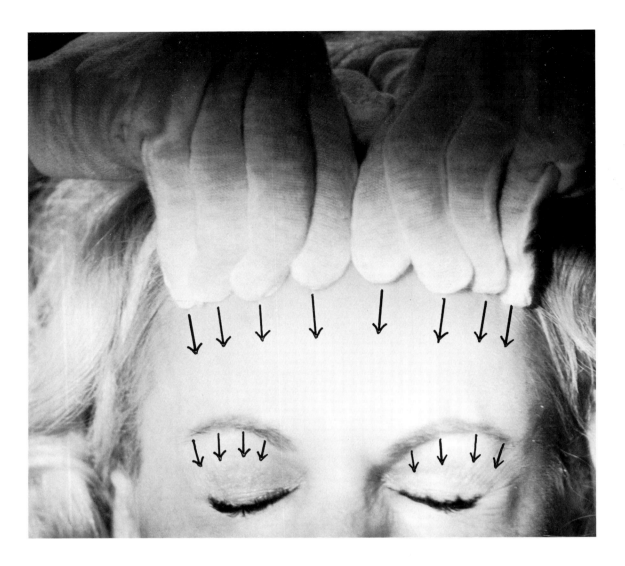

Step 4. Hold the skin tight in this position against the underlying bone. This is now your resistance.

Step 5. Against this resistance first try to move the eyebrows downward, then try to move the forehead skin down out of the resistance, and last, close your eyes tightly.

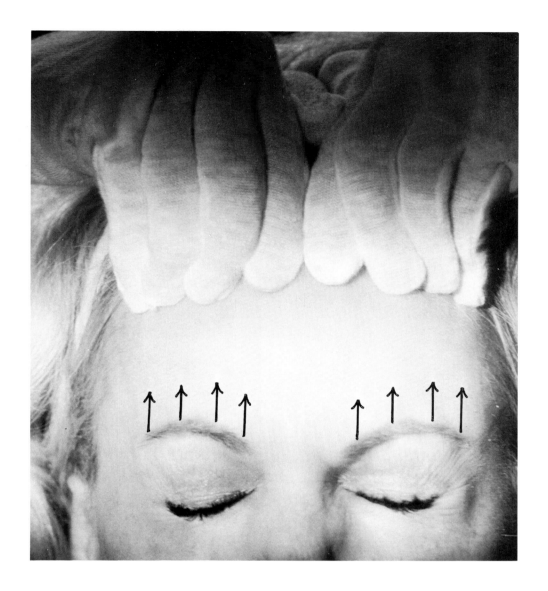

Step 6. Consciously return muscles to starting position.

Step 7. Remove finger resistance.

Purpose: Expanding designated muscles freely and without tension in their fullest range, approximately ¼ to ½ inch.

Note: Resistance must not be moved throughout this exercise. Do not scowl during the muscle movements — move muscles straight down.

Refer: Page (58). - AIM: 5 steps with eyebrows and 10 more steps with forehead muscles, holding eyes tight for 6 counts; return muscles in 10 steps.

Frequency: Once a day 3 times in succession. Hands must be removed and results observed after each performance.

Results: A correct performance will show immediate results. However, frowning must be avoided in order to keep the lines out.

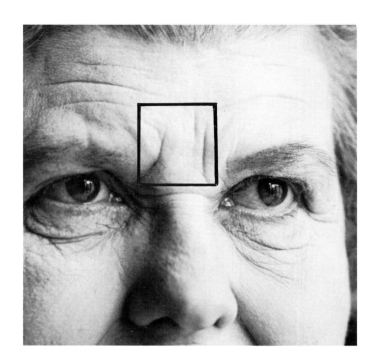

Scowl

Like horizontal lines on the forehead, scowl lines will show up in a face only if forced to appear. Scowl lines are muscles which have been formed into lines by the habit of pulling the brows together.

Since those lines are not an aging fault — young people can have them too — their removal does not give you a younger face but it does, indeed, give a friendlier and more attractive expression.

ENCOURAGEMENT: . . . *I am 28 years and was able to remove my vertical frown lines with one exercise. Thanks to your instruction. Now I am working hard to keep them out.*

B. C., Pasadena, Calif.

To Remove Vertical Lines Between The Eyebrows.

PRELIMINARY PRACTICE:
(to isolate and to gain awareness of the scowling muscles)

- - - Apply a thick coating of Senta Maria Runge's Exercise Cremé over the area involved in scowling.

- - - Sitting or standing position. Look into mirror.

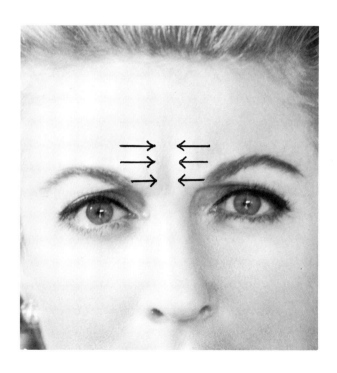

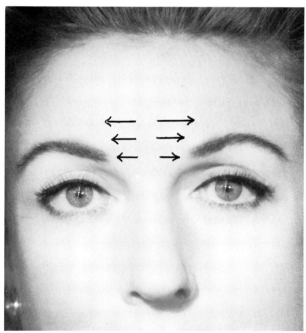

a) In 10-12 even steps, one step to each count, move your brows together to form your habitual scowl line(s).

b) In 10-12 even steps return the brows to their starting position.

Note: Do this PRELIMINARY PRACTICE only a few times then discontinue and proceed with the ISOMETRIC EXERCISE. As cruel as it may look, you must witness each step in your mirror!

Purpose: To move the designated muscles evenly and in their fullest range into YOUR habitual scowl line(s).

- - - Perform only after you have mastered the PRELIMINARY PRACTICE.

- - - Sitting position. Look into mirror.

- - - Scowl exercise object needed.

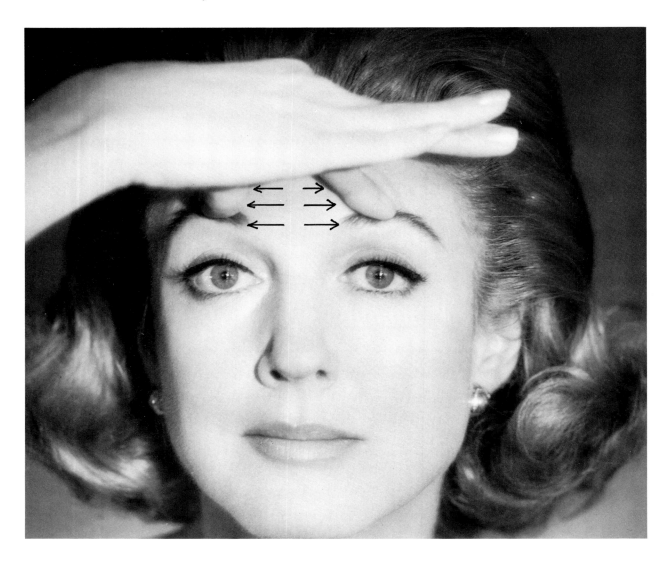

Step 1. Smooth line(s) between eyebrows by pushing the eyebrows apart with fingers as much as possible.

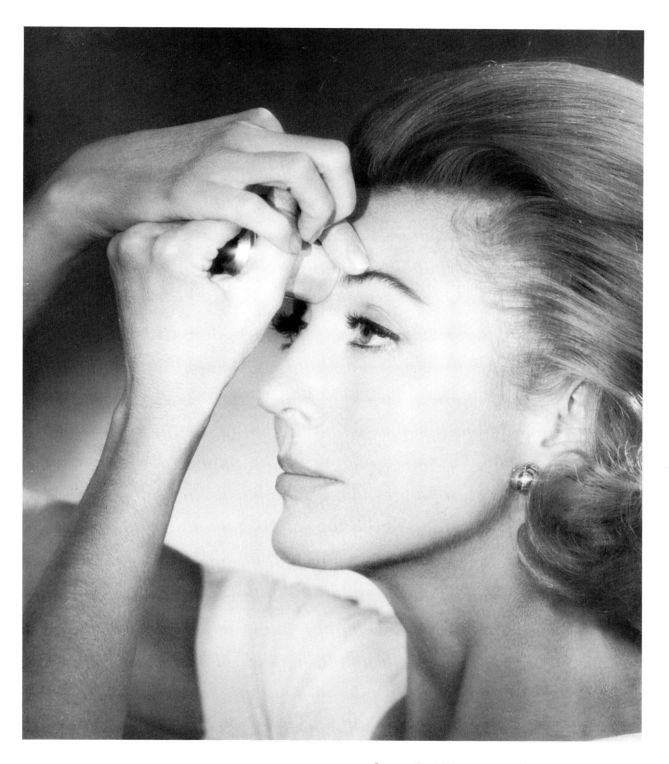

Step 2. With the other hand place object over the smoothed out scowl line area.

Step 3. For resistance press object firm and flat against underlying bone.

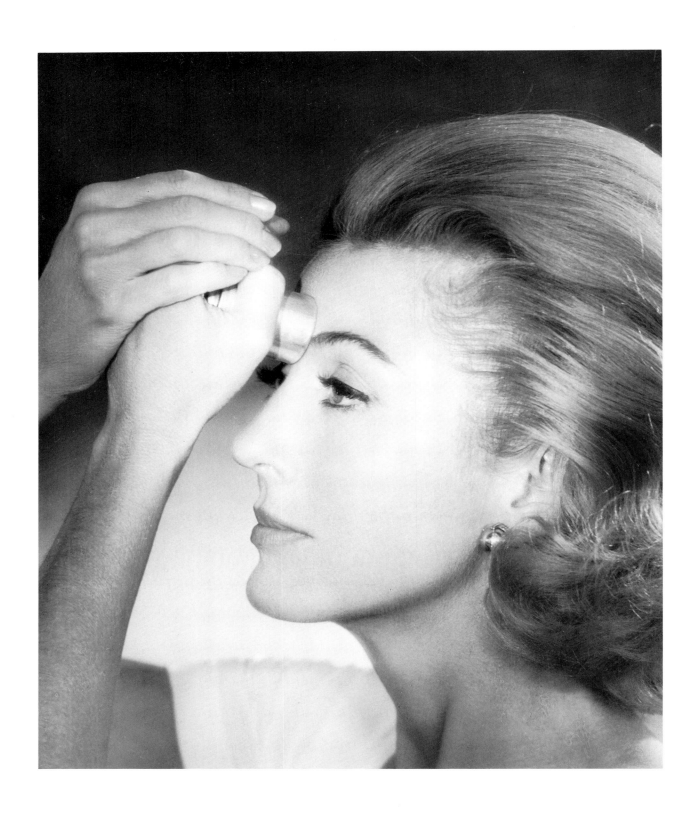

Step 4. Now remove fingers which held the eyebrows apart and use both hands for firm pressure.

Step 5. Against this pressure (resistance) try to scowl (see picture) as you have practiced WITH EYES LOOKING STRAIGHT AHEAD — DO NOT LOOK DOWN!

Step 6. Return muscles in 10 steps to starting position.

Step 7. Release and remove resistance.

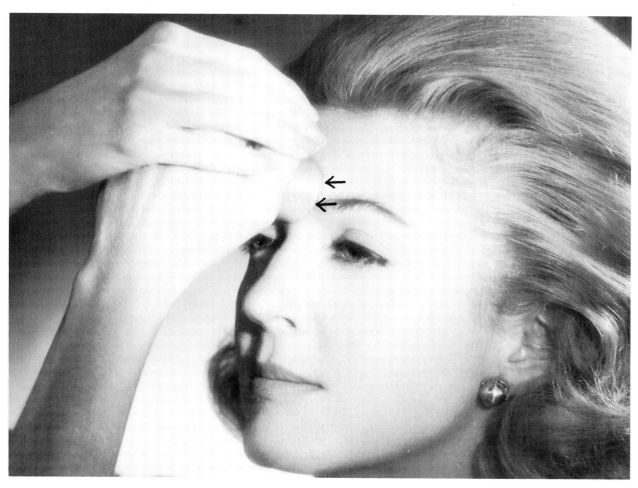

Refer: Page (58). - AIM: 15 steps; return muscles in 10 steps.

Frequency: Once a day 3 times in succession or until line(s) completely disappeared from the contour.

Results: A correct performance may cause the line(s) to disappear or at least to improve greatly. However, to keep the line(s) out scowling must be avoided.

Purpose: Expanding designated muscles freely and to their fullest range.

Note: As soon as you have learned to do the isometric exercise correctly, coat your scowl line area slightly with Senta Maria Runge's Exercise Cremé and place a tissue napkin between the object and creamed skin to avoid slipping. This will help to remove scowl line(s) etched into the skin. The exercise removes the line(s) only from the contour.

EXERCISE No. 10-A

ISOMETRIC EXERCISE:

To Remove Vertical Lines (Scowl Lines) On Forehead & Between Eyebrows.

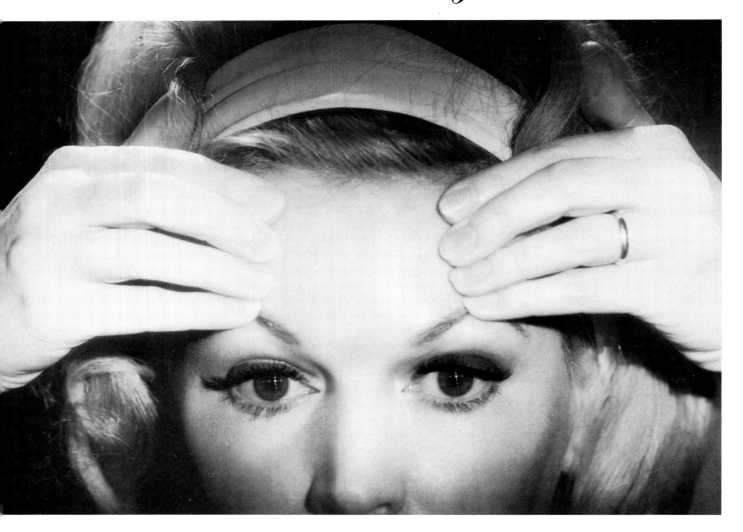

- - - Perform only after you have mastered the PRELIMINARY PRACTICE.

- - - Wear cosmetic gloves to avoid slipping.

Step 1. Place your four fingers of each hand in an even row close behind YOUR last vertical forehead line. Small fingers hold in the eyebrows.

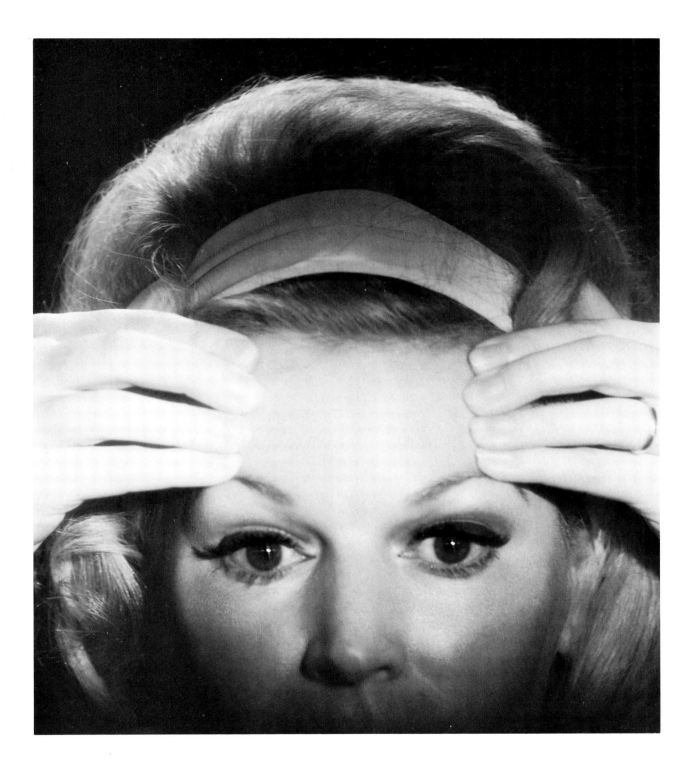

Step 2. Push forehead skin, including eyebrows, outward to smooth out every vertical line on forehead.

Step 3. Hold fingers tight against underlying bone for resistance.

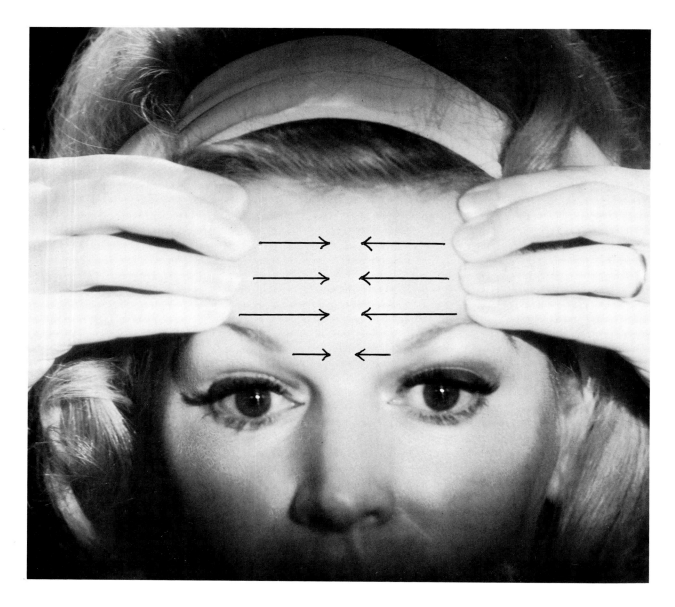

Step 4. Against this resistance try to move your forehead muscles into your habitual line(s) in 5 steps, WITH EYES LOOKING STRAIGHT AHEAD — DO NOT LOOK DOWN.

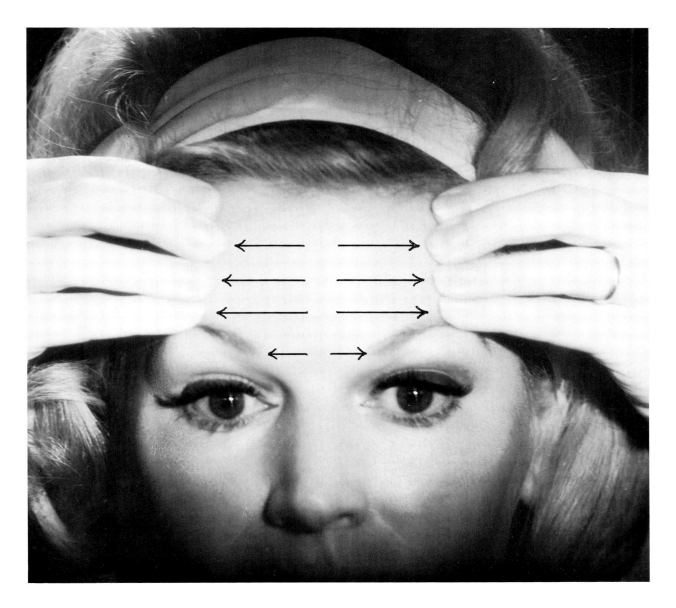

Step 5. Consciously return muscles to starting position.

Step 6. Now release and remove resistance.

Purpose: Expanding designated muscles freely in their fullest range.

Note: Resistance must not move during muscle movements.

Refer: Page (58). - AIM: 15 steps; return muscles in 10 steps.

Frequency: Once a day 3 times in succession or until lines have completely disappeared from the contour.

Results: A correct performance may cause the line(s) to disappear or at least to improve greatly. However, to keep the line(s) from reappearing, scowling must be avoided.

Upper Eyelids.

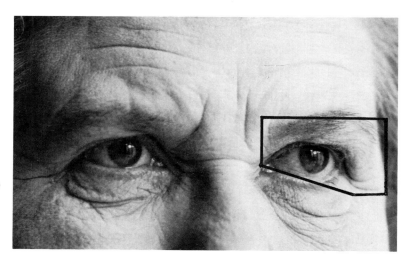

The upper eyelid muscles next to the upper cheek muscles are a means of determining the youth or aging of a face. The muscles constituting the upper eyelids may either atrophy (waste away) or simply elongate. Upper eyelids falling behind the eyeballs usually indicate atrophy, whereas an overlapping muscle-skin usually reveals elongation of the muscles involved. Of course, we see only the skin loose and hanging, however, it is the muscle structure constituting our eyelids that has stretched. The skin consequently has to go with the muscles. By the same token, the skin will shorten and return with the muscles through these exercises.

Those having been born with low positioned brows or overlapping upper eyelids usually have inherited this particuar muscle structure which cannot be changed through exercises.

The lowering of the eyebrows due to the collapse of the upper eyelid muscles, causes our eyes to appear smaller and distorts, a la da Vinci, the proportioning of the face.

ENCOURAGEMENT: . . . *I have had puffy, lax upper eyelids, and now they have taken on new life.*

B. P., Huntington Park, Calif.

To Lift Droopy Eyebrows & To Firm Slack Overhanging Upper Eyelids

PRELIMINARY PRACTICE:
(to isolate and to gain awareness of the eyebrow and upper eyelid muscles)

- - - Sitting or standing position. Mirror in front.

- - - Apply thick coating of Senta Maria Runge's Exercise Cremé above eyebrows and on forehead.

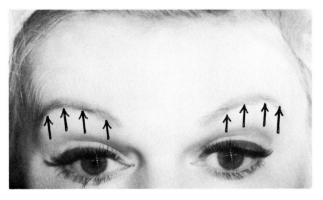

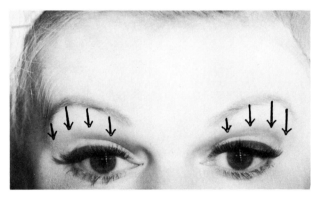

a) In 5 even steps move both eyebrows upward as far as possible. The point of possibility is when you see no more overlapping on your upper eyelids.

b) Consciously return eyebrows in 5 even steps.

Purpose: Moving designated muscles to their fullest range, approximately ½ to ¾ inch, without tension or help by surrounding muscles.

Refer: Page (58). - AIM: 10 steps; return muscles in 10 steps.

Frequency: As often as you wish until you have conquered your AIM.

Note: In particular, pay attention to the sides of the lids and brows, since those muscles are thinner and more difficult to move. The leading muscles in the movement must be the weakest ones, as indicated by the droopiest muscle skin.

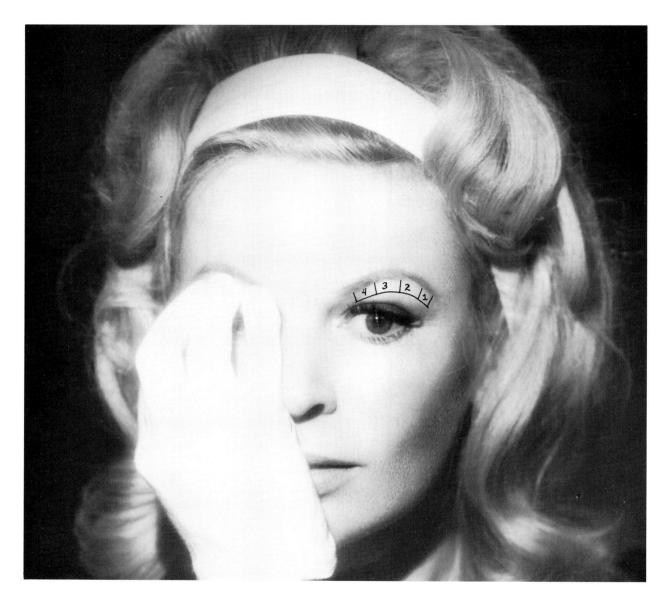

- - - Sitting or standing position; look in mirror.

- - - Cosmetic gloves may be used to avoid slipping; elbows on table.

Step 1. With forehead relaxed, apply resistance to both of your natural brows from beneath by placing your four finger points under each brow at the location indicated on picture. The finger points must be directly on the brow but not in it.

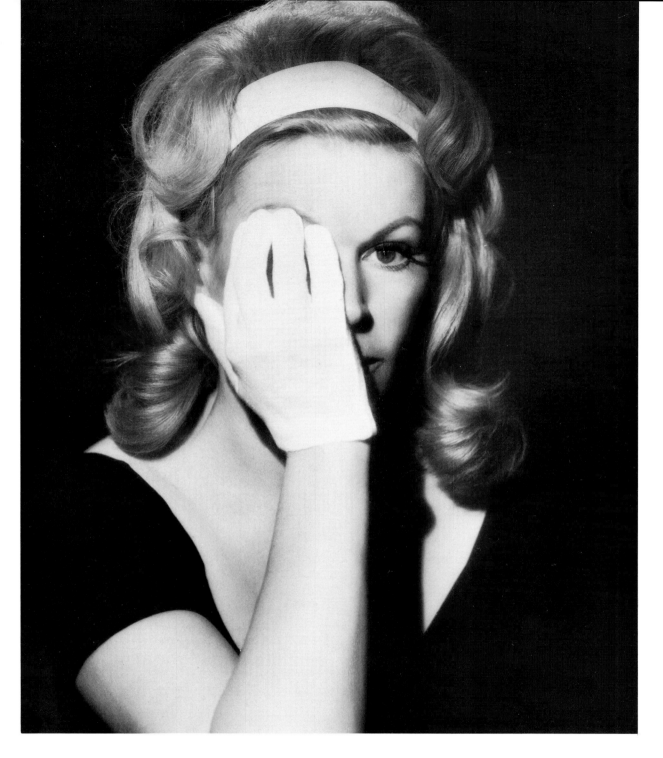

Step 2. With fingers push both eye-brows upward to their youthful, original position, and hold them there firmly as a resistance.

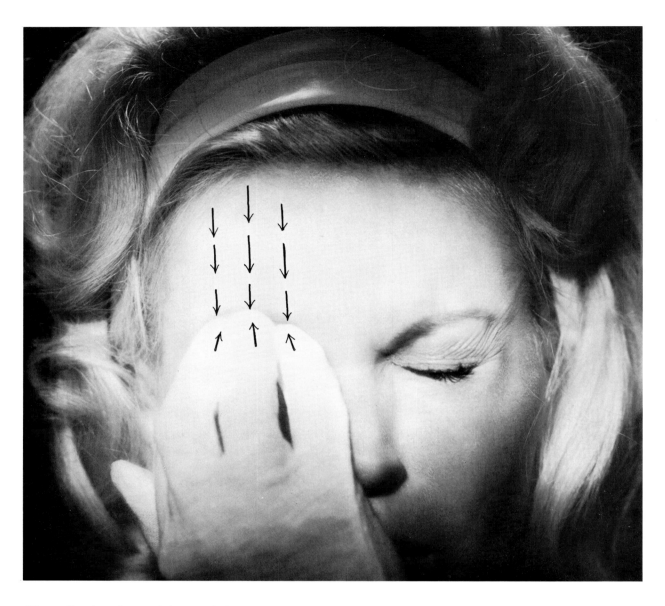

Step 3. Against this resistance try to move your brows down in gradual repetitious attempts; then try to move your forehead down from the very top and at last close your eyes tight.

Step 4. Return muscles to starting position.

Step 5. Remove finger resistance.

Purpose: Expanding designated muscles freely and without tension to their fullest range.

Note: It is important that you do not look downward but straight ahead while you move the muscles out of the eyebrow and forehead. The aim must be to move the muscles out of eyebrow and forehead STRAIGHT down and not inward as for scowling. Concentrate on the weakest spot and on the sides of the brows. Do not deceive yourself by tensing up in the lower eyelids instead of actually trying to move the brows down. The resistance, however, has to be immobile.

Refer: Page (58). - AIM: 10-12 steps, closing eyes tightly for 6 counts; return muscles in 10 steps.

Frequency: Once a day 3 times in succession. Hands must be removed and results observed after each performance.

Results: A correct performance will show a drastic lift of the brows. In areas where you do not see the brows lifted, you either have not held the resistance or you have not moved the muscles in this area.

Suggestions: Puffiness in the upper eyelids may indicate fatty tissues or fluid. For fluid see your doctor. Fatty tissues can be removed successfully through plastic surgery.

Lower Eyelids

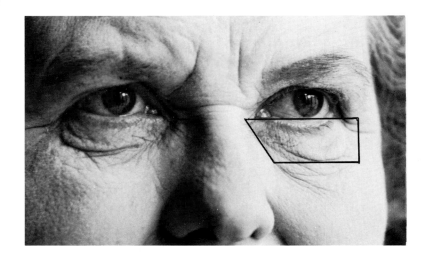

The muscles in the lower eyelids elongate about half an inch between the ages of 21 and 60. This is understandable when we consider how much strain is put on these tiny, delicate muscle tissues. Also, the skin in this area is extremely fine and sensitive. Here too, as with the upper eyelids, we can see only the skin, loose and hanging, adapting to its muscle foundation. Every line you see in your lower eyelid is a muscle attached to the skin which has elongated. The lower eyelid may also appear more sunken-in with the passage of years, due to the loss of fatty tissue in the skin, which unfortunately cannot be regained. A sunken-in "tired look" in that area caused by tired muscles due to lack of circulation however, can be improved miraculously through my exercise.

Circles around the eyes which existed before muscular relaxation, cannot be removed by exercising. Those troubled with puffiness in the eye area due to a sinus or allergy condition will find my exercise utmost beneficial. The mentioned condition causes lack of circulation in the eye area, thus permitting fluid (edema) to collect in the tissues. Do you awaken sometimes — most likely after a long sleep — with puffy eyelids? In this case it is also the slow circulation during your prolonged sleep that permits fluid to inhabit the tissues in the eyelid region. The eye exercises will help you get rid of this distracting puffiness.

ENCOURAGEMENT: . . .

. . . Have had many compliments in the past few weeks. I am 44 years old and people are telling me I don't look older than 32. Another said my eyes were so bright. Have been erasing wrinkles like mad.

E. H., Covina, Calif.

To Fill Out Hollowness & To Remove Circles (Due To Tiredness) & To Remove Lines.

PRELIMINARY PRACTICE:
(to isolate and to gain awareness of the lower eyelid muscles)

- - - Sitting or standing position.

- - - Apply a thick layer of Senta Maria Runge's Exercise Cremé around lower eyelids and in the crow's feet area.

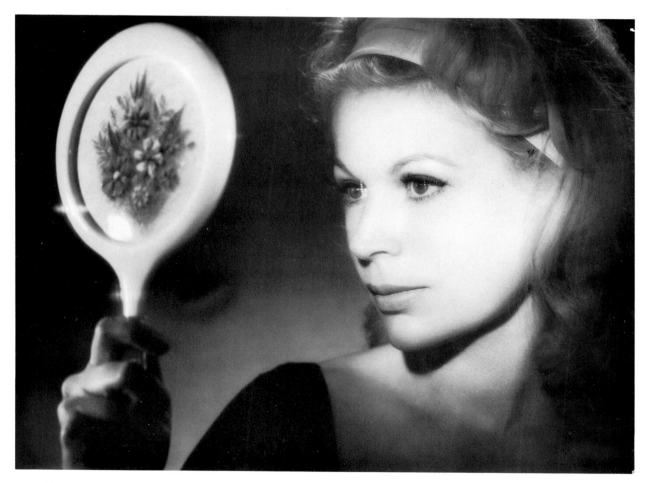

a) Hold mirror in hand and look straight into the mirror in front of you.

b) Then lower head somewhat so that you have to look up slightly to see your eyes in the mirror. DO NOT raise eyebrows.

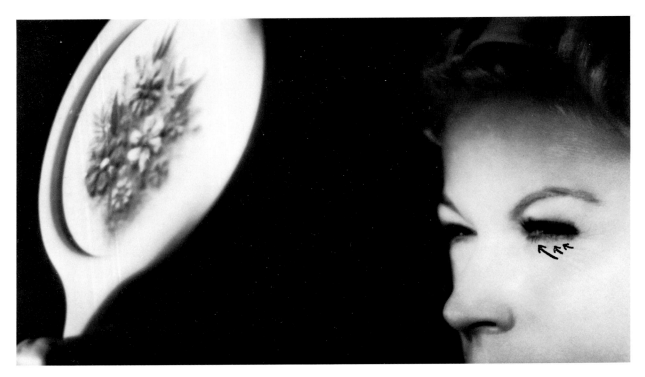

c) In even movements raise lower eyelids upward to the center (blinking).

d) Notice that by your will you can move each wrinkle individually or all together, hence every wrinkle in the lower eyelid is a muscle. Please also observe that every one of those wrinkles performs diagonally upward toward the nose.

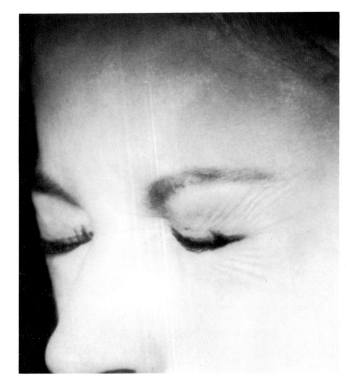

e) Close both eyelids in center position tightly and hold tightness for 3 counts. After each count breathe deeply.

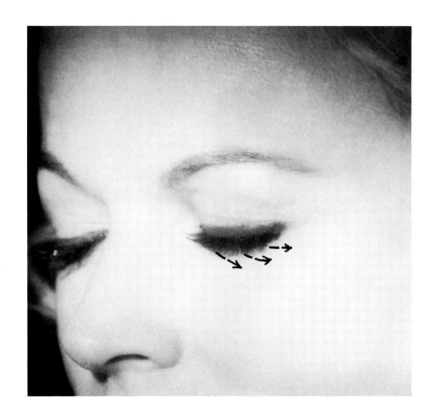

f) With closed eyelids return lower eyelid muscles (like slowly falling asleep).

Purpose: Moving designated muscles freely and without tension to their fullest range.

Note: Do not push the lower lid muscles with your cheek muscles.

Refer: Page (58). - AIM: 10 steps and keep eyes closed for 3 counts; return muscles in 10 steps.

Frequency: Once or twice a day 3 times in succession.

I S O M E T R I C
E X E R C I S E :

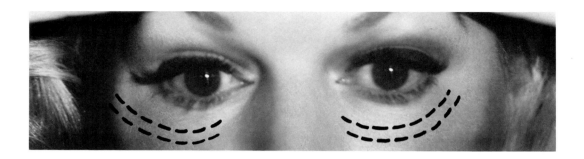

- - - Do not attempt unless PRELIM-INARY PRACTICE has been mastered.

- - - Sitting position. Mirror standing in front of you.

- - - Work on both lower eyelids simultaneously.

- - - Apply Senta Maria Runge's Exercise Creme around lower eyelids.

- - - Lie tissue paper over creamed area to avoid slipping off with the resistance.

- - - Rest elbows on table.

Step 1. Fit lower part of hands (See diagram.) flat and carefully — so as not to push skin — on *the edge* of the bone below eyes.

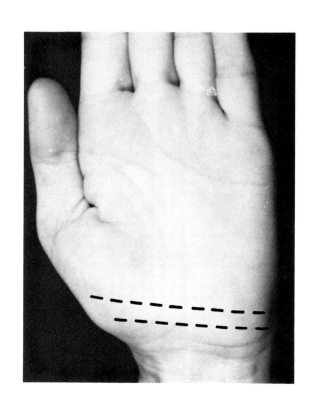

Step 2. Press against edge of bone for the count of six. Pressure should be gradually from soft to hard. Now hold pressure firm and steady for resistance.

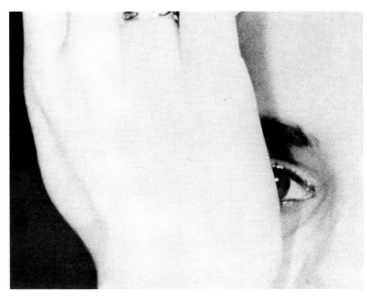

Step 3. Against this resistance, gradually raise lower eyelids upwards as you have practised in your Preliminary. Your mind should follow the muscle movements — a step to a count.

Step 4. At the center of the eyes, close eyes tightly and take a deep breath.

Step 5. Return lower eyelids to starting position and open eyes.

Step 6. Release resistance and remove hands.

Step 7. Evaluate results in your mirror and adjust if necessary the hand placement for the consequent application.

PURPOSE: Expanding designated muscles freely to their fullest range.

CAUTION: If the area below the eyes shows considerable puffiness due to fatty tissue or fluid retention, do not apply this resistance exercise, but the Preliminary only. The Isometric, however, may be most beneficial for slight puffiness resulting from fluid retention (edema) due to lack of circulation in that area.

NOTE: The skin in the lower eyelid area is very thin, therefore, moving the sensitive skin by hands has to be avoided. The benefit from the exercise is great if precisely done, however, slipping off with the resistance or pushing with the hands has to be avoided. Every hand is different and one has to experiment to see which part of the hands fits best on the edge of the bone. If hands or fingers do not fit, take them straight off until you find the right position. Use even pressure during the exercise.

REFER: Page 58 — A I M 8 steps upward and keep eyes tightly closed for six counts, returning muscles in ten steps.

FREQUENCY: Daily — three times in succession. Fingers must be removed and results observed after every performance. Apply Exercise Creme before EACH exercise application.

RESULTS: If performed correctly, the results from each performance are instantaneously miraculous.

Crow's Feet

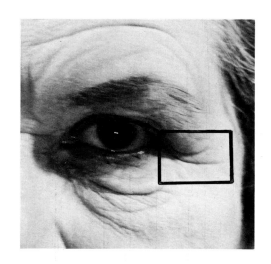

Crow's feet are expression lines caused by the habit of squinting. The lines may be only "skin deep" and, therefore, can be ironed out of the skin by the principle of ironing a wrinkled cloth. However, if the crow's feet have inhabited the contour, then we have to restore the muscles involved through an isometric exercise. An overlapping upper eyelid may also appear in the form of crow's feet. However, since these particular lines are caused by elongated upper lid muscles it can be eliminated only by exercising the cause.

ENCOURAGEMENT: *. . . I am amazed at the way the crow's feet and wrinkles around my eyes are disappearing already. It just doesn't seem possible at my age (66 years) but I am so encouraged and will keep right on with it.*

G. M. P., Los Angeles, Calif.

. . . How could I explain this to my employer? Today I stayed home from work because I felt ill. I was happy to have had the opportunity to watch your TV program. Tomorrow, I am returning to work without crow's feet and a fresh and young look around my eyes which my employer has never seen on me before.

B. T., Los Angeles, Calif.

Iron Out Crow's Feet Lines From The Skin.

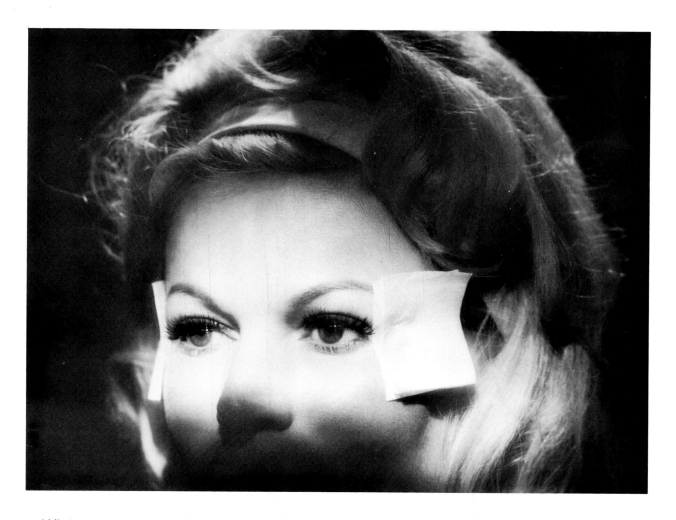

Wherever we have a line or lines in the skin (not referring to contour lines caused by collapsed or misformed muscles) we can iron those lines out of the skin by the principle of ironing a wrinkled cloth.

- - - Sitting position; elbows resting on table. Look into mirror.

- - - Apply Senta Maria Runge's Exercise Creme over the crow's feet lines. Place a tissue napkin over the creamed area.

a) The wrinkled skin is our cloth which we have moistened with the exercise creme.

b) The ironing board is a firm bone underneath the wrinkled skin.

c) The iron itself is a flat and firm pressure by our hands.

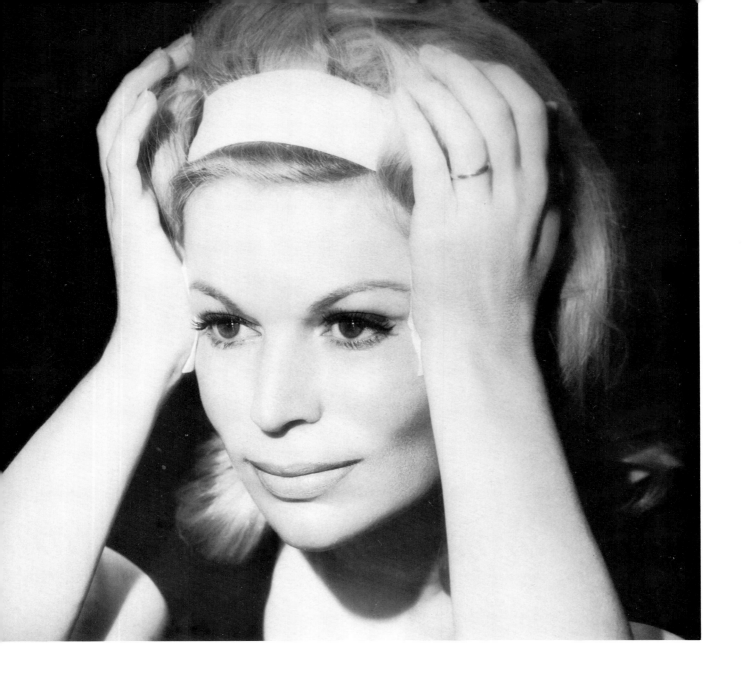

Step 1. Lift eyebrows somewhat up and place flat part of hands or thumb beside eyes, covering the wrinkled skin area including the edge of the bone.

Step 2. Press from soft increasingly to utmost firmness while you count slowly to 15.

Step 3. Release pressure gradually to the count of 10.

Frequency: Once a day 3 times in succession.

Results: If done properly, lines will be diminished. Remaining lines indicate insufficient flat or firm pressure in this area. Treat such lines separately.

Note: Squinting, of course, has to be avoided! What lasting good is it to iron out wrinkles from your garment when you sit down again and put them back in?

To Remove Crow's Feet From The Contour

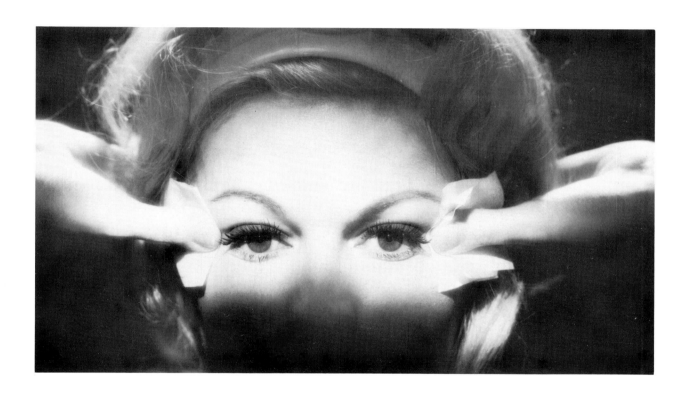

- - - Do not attempt unless PRELIMI-NARY PRACTICE on page (166) has been mastered.

- - - Sitting position. Look into mirror.

- - - Apply Senta Maria Runge's Exercise Creme on skin in crow's feet area. Tissue napkin (cut in 1½ inch square) covering the creamed area to avoid slipping.

Step 1. Lift eyebrows up and fit tip of thumbs or palm of hands flat against the bone beside the eyes, including the edge of this bone.

Step 2. Press from soft increasingly to utmost firmness for 5 counts and keep this position for resistance.

Step 3. Release eyebrows.

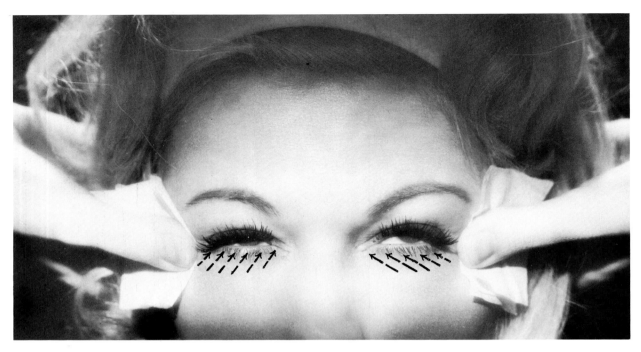

Step 4. Against this resistance lift
lower eyelids slowly to the
center as you have practiced in
the PRELIMINARY PRACTICE.
a) while looking up
b) without frowning

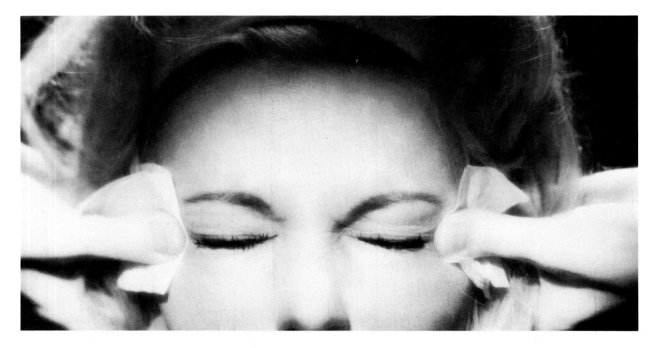

Step 5. Close eyes tightly at center
and keep them closed for 3
counts.

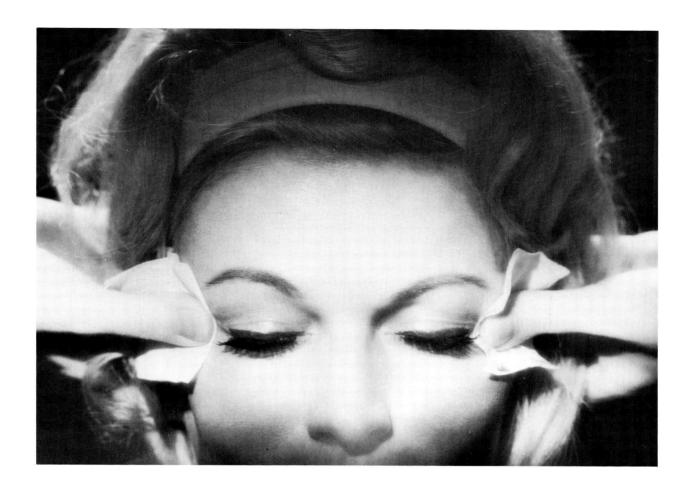

Step 6. With closed eyes, return muscles downward.

Step 7. Now release and remove resistance.

Purpose: Expanding designated muscles freely and to their fullest range without tension or help by other muscles.

Note: Check that you do not scowl during muscle performance.

Refer: Page (58). - AIM: 20 steps, keep eyes tightly closed for 6 steps; return muscles in 10 steps.

Frequency: Once a day 3 times in succession. Hands must be removed and results observed after each performance.

Results: If performed correctly the results from each performance are instantaneously miraculous! A remaining line indicates that you either have not resisted this particular muscle or you have not moved it.

EXERCISE No. 14

ISOMETRIC EXERCISE:

Combined Eye Exercise:

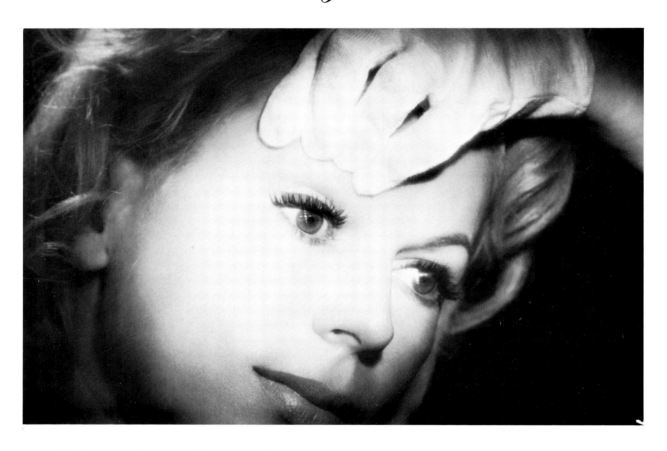

- - - Sitting position, elbow resting on table. Look into mirror.

- - - Apply Senta Maria Runge's Exercise Creme and tissue napkin to lower eyelids.

- - - Apply only after you have mastered ISOMETRIC EXERCISE NO. 12 and NO. 13.

- - - Wear cosmetic glove on hand holding eyebrow.

- - - Can be done on one side at a time only. When exercising on right side of the face, wear glove on left hand.

Step 1. With fingertips of left hand lift the right eyebrow upward and hold this position for firm resistance. (For correct finger position refer to exercise No. 11, page 159). Skin underneath resistance must be evenly taut.

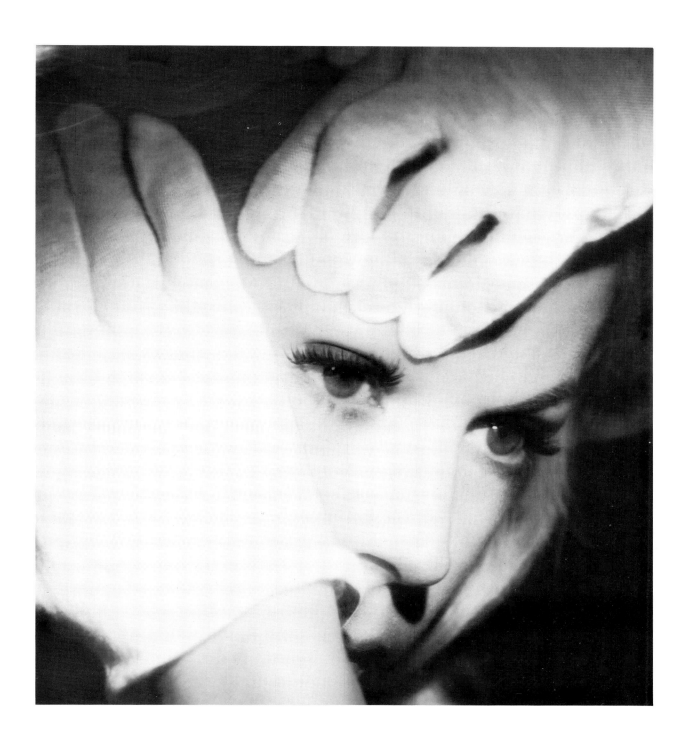

Step 2. Resist lower eyelid and crow's feet muscles by pressing muscle skin in this area against the bone underneath. For firm and steady pressure apply part of hand you used for exercise No. 12.

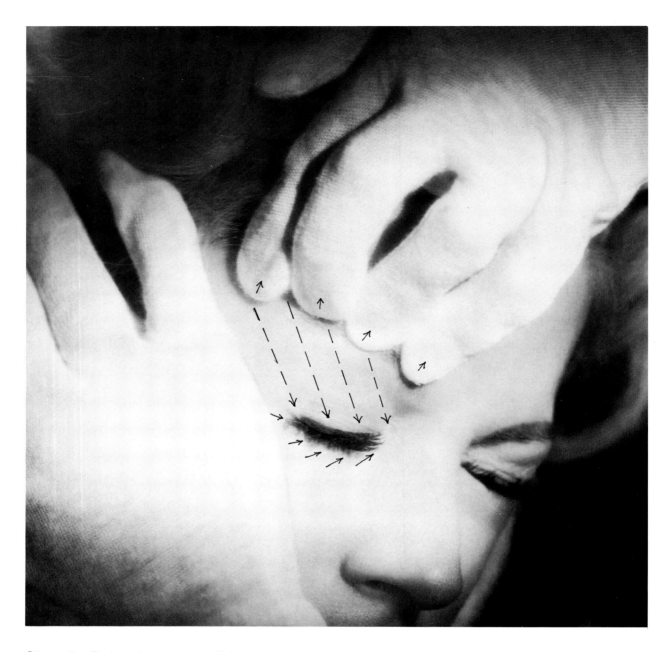

Step 3. Raise lower eyelid upward to center slowly for 10 counts (as practiced previously).

Step 4. Close eye very tightly in center position.

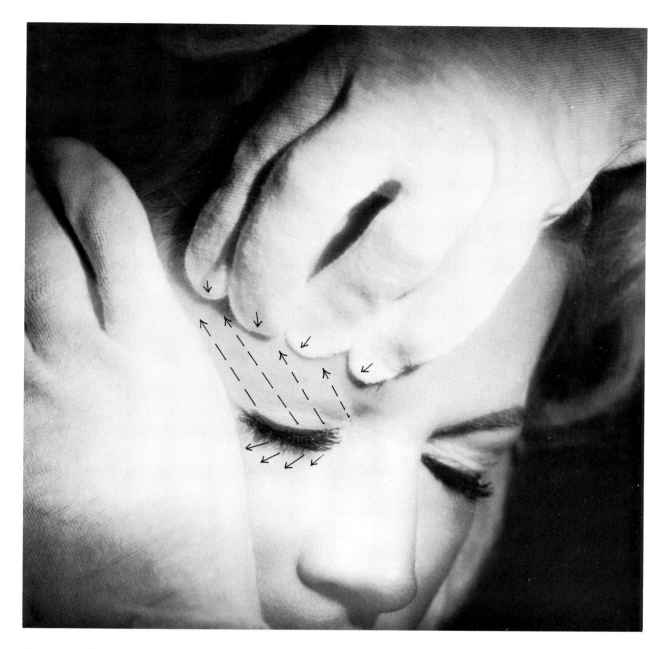

Step 5. Slowly return muscles for 10 steps.

Step 6. Remove resistance.

Purpose: Expanding designated muscles freely and to their fullest range, this includes the muscles of the lower eyelids, crow's feet and upper eyelids.

Note: Resistance must be held steady throughout the exercise.

Refer: Page (58). - AIM: 10 steps with eyes tightly closed for 6 counts; return muscles in 10 steps.

Frequency: Once a day 3 times in succession. Hands must be removed and results observed after each performance.

Results: If performed correctly, the eyebrow must look lifted and the lower eyelid refreshed from each performance.

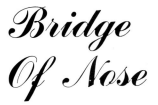

Bridge Of Nose

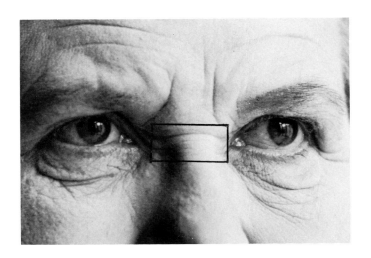

Lines across the bridge of the nose are largely expression lines which inhabit the contour from knitting the brows.

To eliminate these lines, the habit of forming them must be broken and the following exercise applied.

ENCOURAGEMENT: . . . *Please note change of name. For the last three years I ordered under the name of Helen Foster, now it is Mrs. Alex Gradney, thanks to your wonderful exercises and products.*

Mrs. A. G., Beverly Hills

ISOMETRIC EXERCISE:

To Remove Lines From Bridge Of Nose

- - - Sitting or standing position. Look into mirror.

- - - Wear cosmetic gloves to avoid slipping.

Step 1. With four fingerpoints hold muscle skin against nose bone right below the bottom wrinkle across the bridge of the nose.

Step 2. Push muscle skin somewhat down and hold this position firm for resistance. Lines must be smoothed away.

Step 3. Gradually try to move the muscle skin out of your resistance.

Step 4. Consciously return muscle skin to starting position.

Step 5. Now release and remove resistance.

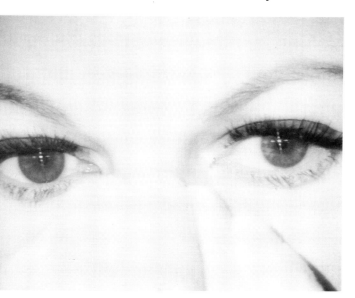

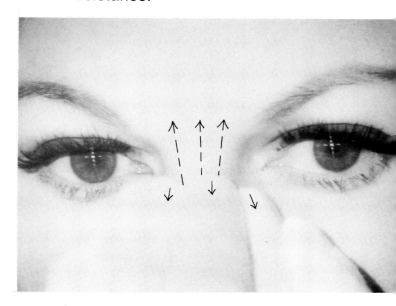

Purpose: Expanding designated muscles freely and to their fullest range without tension or help by other muscles.

Note: Resistance must never move during exercise. Watch that you do not move the eyebrows upward which would cause you to frown.

Refer: Page (58). - AIM: 10 steps; return muscles in 10 steps.

Frequency: Once a day 3-4 times in succession.

Results: If performed correctly some results must show after a few exercise applications.

FACE-EX

This implement was born out of the desire to reduce the time of exercising, to simplify the performance, and to increase optimum beneficial results. Face-Ex became the answer. It took several engineers, in co-operation with plastic surgeons, three years to develop this now so simple solution. Face-Ex is not a machine but an implement that replaces our finger resistance and provides adequate resistance with the most gentle grip even to the strongest cheek muscles.

Its ability to resist one full inch of muscle flesh per application enables one to combine Exercise No. 6 for Pouch, No. 6 for Upper Cheeks, and No. 2 for Jowls, into O N E exercise. Consequently, one particular resistance with Face-Ex enables us to perform an isometric exercise by which we

- - - remove folds above laugh line

- - - fill out hollow and lift droopy upper cheeks

- - - remove pouches beside the chin

- - - lift droopy mouth corners

- - - remove jowls

By studying the muscle face on page 80, you will note that it is mostly the Zygomaticus and partly the Labii muscle (identified in my diagram on page 125 as Muscle Section 1 & 2) which is responsible for the five above mentioned conditions.

Exercising with Face-Ex is fool-proof, and absolutely no damage to skin or muscles can occur, since it cannot slip when applied correctly. However, I do not advise the use of Face-Ex **before** one has learned Exercise No. 6 (Muscle Section 1 & 2) with finger resistance to the point that one obtains results from every exercise application. It is easier to **work** with Face-Ex only if one knows how to do the exercises (muscle movements) correctly. It is however easier to **learn** the exercises with finger resistance because one has more feeling of one's flesh when held by fingers, as compared to being held by an implement.

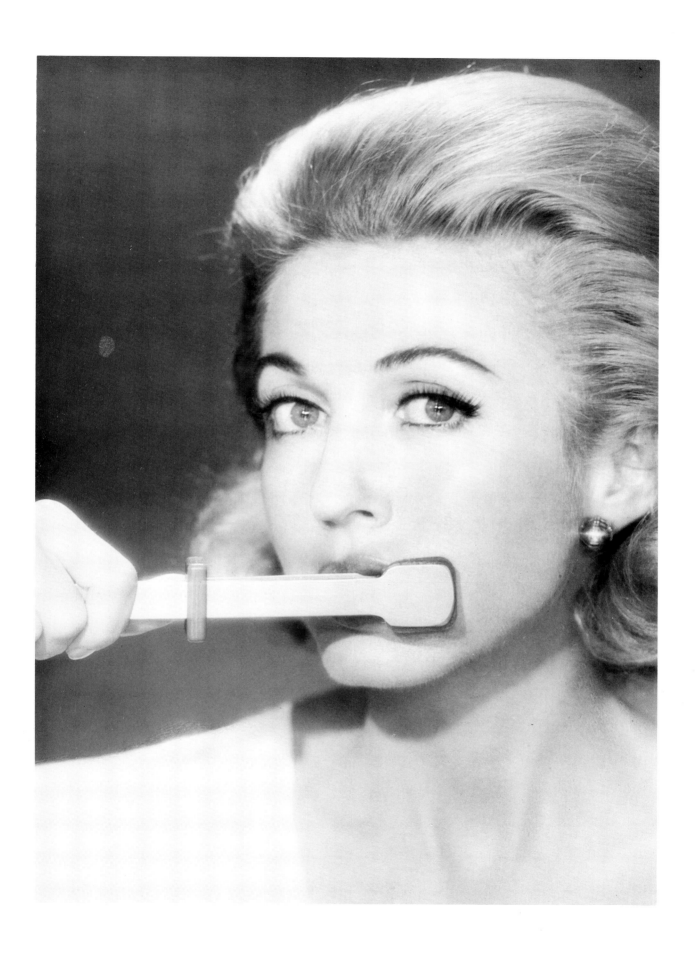

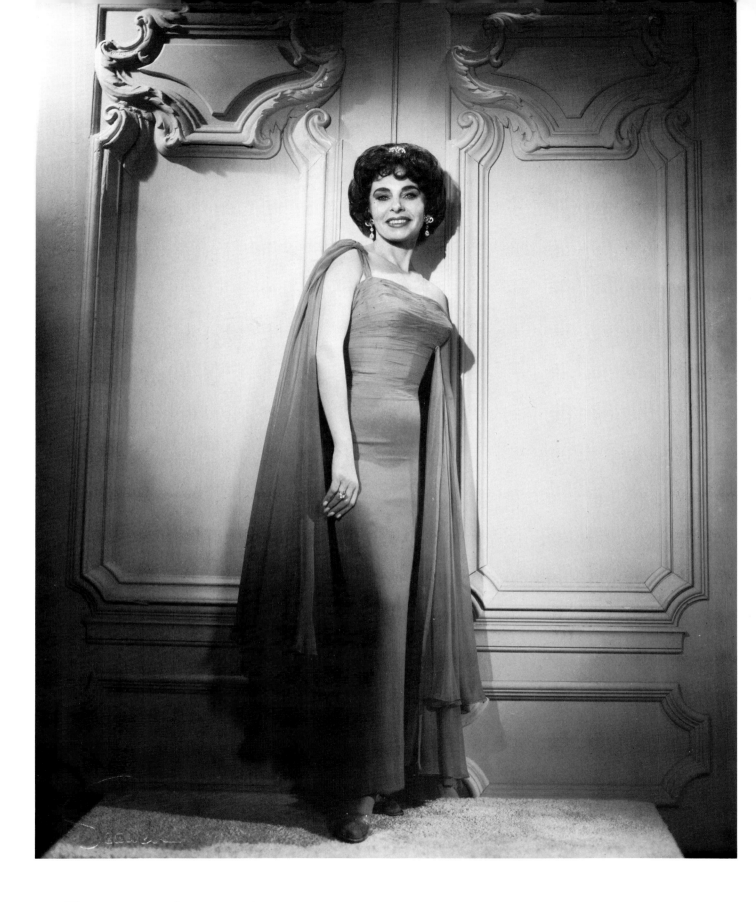

Senta Maria Rungé

FACE LIFTING BY EXERCISE
KTLA-TV, HOLLYWOOD

EXCERPTS FROM TESTIMONIALS

. . . For the first time I have watched my mother doing the exercises advocated on your program. She has been doing them for several weeks and our whole family has noticed the improvement. Although I am only 16, I would like to begin them in time to completely avoid wrinkles on my face.

A. G., Los Angeles California

. . . Having been a motion picture actress, now retired, I have used many, many brands of creams and oils on my skin, but never have I come across one that makes my skin feel so alive and fresh. I am getting satisfactory results from the exercises, even my husband notices an improvement and encourages me to exercise each day.

(confidential)

. . . Being a Doctor's wife I have had access to all sorts of hypo allergenic products. Most of these are about as effective as water. Your creams are positively in a class by themselves.

Mrs. K., Pasadena, California

. . . Thousands and thousands of women could not help but be happy when they could see the results of your cosmetics and exercises. This could not help but bring a chain reaction of happiness in the home — also outside the home — for how could any woman have unkind thoughts or feelings for any one when she is so happy looking at herself and seeing the years gone from her face through the use of your creams and exercises.

Mrs. A. H. M.

. . . I bless the day I watched you as I have learned so much that has helped me now in years to come. As far as I am concerned your facial exercises were sent from heaven from you to us.

R. D. P., Granada Hills, Calif.

. . . You are solving my problem! I have been 25 pounds overweight for several years. I am now 40 plus a few years old. I have been so discouraged by my "droopy puss" that I would toss my diet out of the window, preferring a plump face and tummy. I started dieting 2 weeks ago, inspired by your specialized exercises — and I am thrilled to say that I have lost my first five pounds and my face has better tone than before. My doctor will love you.

A. W., Sepulveda, Calif.

. . . I have a copy of your book "Face Lifting by Exercise" and am following your T.V. program and am most enthusiastic about the results I am having. This is the best thing that has happened to me for a long time! I want to pass the news along to others.

S. W.

. . . I receive the most extravagant compliments about my appearance. I am 41½ and people always guess me to be 31 or 26 and recently some lady whom I had met several times said she had thought I was about 23. Isn't that something? Thank you for this wonderful system of facial rejuvenation which you have revealed.

B. C., Woodland Hills, California

. . . My mother and I watch your program faithfully and have benefited very much from your exercises.

H. D., Torrance, California

. . . I have only been with your television program a short while, and the improvement in my face is almost unbelievable. Thanks for giving me a complete new lease on life, for I had given up hope until I found you!

Mrs. C. R. B., Covina, California

. . . I just passed my 42nd birthday and people tell me that I look like I am about 26. Thanks to you.

Mrs. L. K., Ventura, California

. . . Your facial exercises have done far more for me the past few months than my 2 facial exercise machines have in years. At 34 I look much younger than I did 8 years ago. Nothing I can say could really express just how grateful I am to you.

S. F. J., St. Paul, Minnesota

. . . I have seen all your models and the miracles you performed on each of them.

M. M., San Pedro, California

. . . Thank you so very much for making life so much more interesting for me. I raised 5 wonderful children and when they married I took a good look at "me" for the first time in 25 years. I found myself looking much older than I should have, but did not know what to do about it. But about that time I tuned in your program "Face Lifting by Exercise" - what a break! It was just what I needed. Your creams are wonderful and a lot more. Your exercises really perform miracles. People are saying to me, "What happened to you." Truly I already look 10 years younger and have just started.

O. R., Big Bear Lake, California

. . . After 3 months I look 35 not 41. My daughter tells me so. I am so grateful!

Mrs. B. J. A., Oceanside, California

. . . You are absolutely heaven sent! I don't know when anything has excited me as much as your program. I will be 56 this year and as far as I was concerned, I looked twice that. The sags and droops were so pronounced that I mentally drooped too. I could exercise and become more supple — keep my weight down — and dress as becomingly as possible — but the droopy face was always the same. One morning I went through all the exercises with you on T.V. while my husband was watching. He expressed great amazement when my jowls practically disappeared right before his eyes. I have noticed many women friends peering at me with searching eyes . . . and now I tell everyone who will listen about you.

Mrs. K., Pasadena, California

. . . You just don't know how much good you are doing for many of us who want to improve the facial appearance.

Mrs. C. D., Oxnard, Calif.

. . . Your wonderful creams and exercises helped minimize bad scars on my neck.

Mrs. C. M. St., Van Nuys, Calif.

. . . There are no words to express my enthusiasm about your program. It would take volumes to even try.

. . . Los Angeles, Calif.

. . . What hope you have given to all women. I cannot bear to think what it would be like never to have discovered your method of regaining a more youthful face and your helpful hints of proper care for the skin.

A. M., Huntington Park, Calif.

. . . Your program is a blessing to so many of us. Your exercises have given me a new lease on life, but being a busy business woman and home maker, your time on T.V. is my only indulgence. I see wonderful improvement in my face. My friends look at me and compliment on how well I am looking. I am quick to tell them about your Face Lifting by Exercise method. I hope to have the opportunity to personally show you my good results, for I am 56 years old and like to take pride in my youthful appearance.

Mrs. T. K., Pacific Palisades, Calif.

. . . May I add my voice to the many singing your praise. Your exercises are the most wonderful Christmas present anyone can ever receive.

J. H., Brea, Calif.

. . . I met a woman a month ago, who had the most beautiful face. She looked about·25 or 26. She told us she was 46 years old. She also told us about your method.

S. H., North Hollywood, Calif.

. . . I am so thrilled with your wonderful program, you are truly heaven sent! God bless you in your work.

Mrs. E. M., Culver City, Calif.

. . . Bless you for coming along with your wonderful method. I am eternally grateful to you.

M. L., Pacoima, Calif.

. . . Your exercises are giving me a real "lift" literally and figuratively. Please, please continue forever.

Mrs. S. L., Los Angeles, Calif.

. . . Words are inadequate to tell you what your exercises and products have done for me - it's really a miracle. To me you deserve a medal for the greatest morale builder in our country. Any woman using your exercises and creams faithfully can watch the years roll off - now what could be better for the morale?

Mrs. A. H. M., Woodland Hills, Calif.

. . . I am so grateful to you for all you have given us and for your wonderful products.

Mrs. T. W., Los Angeles, Calif.

. . . I am so thankful to have found your program with the gift you have for humanity.

A. S., La Jolla, California

. . . Please note change of name. For the last three years I ordered under the name of Helen Foster, now it is Mrs. Alex Gradney, thanks to your wonderful exercises and products.

Mrs. A. G., Beverly Hills

THE FOLLOWING EXCERPTS ARE IN REPLY TO A QUESTION-
NAIRE WE SENT ALONG WITH THE INTRODUCTION OF OUR
C-PRODUCTS. (All original testimonials are on file.)

Q. WHAT RESULTS HAVE YOU OBTAINED FROM USING THE C-
PRODUCTS?

A. *Fantastic! Closed my pores and gives my skin a firm, youthful appearance.
It is beyond description!*

F.S., Miami, Fl.

A. *It closed my enlarged pores and made my skin look more youthful.*

A.F., Indiana

A. *Due to a severe case of acne, when young, my skin was left with tiny scars
and enlarged pores (cheeks). Without much hope, I decided to try your
C-3 Cream and Lotion. To my great surprise and joy, I find my skin much
softer and the scars and enlarged pores receding. Very satisfactory!*

Mrs. W.A.W., Georgia

A. *I am absolutely thrilled at the results.*

P.R.B., North Carolina

A. *My skin never has been so smooth and clear and moist.*

M.A., Boulder, Co.

A. *Excellent! My skin is much clearer and tighter. The C-3 Lotion I use over the
make-up makes my skin glow.*

Mrs. C.H., New York

A. *If this refining of the pores continues, yours will be the first product that has
been able to accomplish this.*

C.P., Nevada

A. *Feels and looks like my own natural moisture.*

A.G., Lakewood, CA.

A. *In my opinion the C-3 Cream & Lotion are excellent products and words cannot express my satisfaction with them.*

I.T., Glendale, Arizona

A. *I have found these products to be extremely effective.*

C.H., New York

A. *I like it very much, along with the application of the C-2 Cream. It leaves my complexion and skin 100% improved over what it was previously. It is not greasy and absorbs well.*

T.R., Denver

A. *After a few days my skin had a beautiful texture, I couldn't believe it.*

Mrs. R.C., Chicago

A. *Much tighter skin — no more acne or breakouts — Fantastic.*

L.K., Skokie

A. *My skin is smooth, silky and looks more alive than it has since I was about 25 years old. My make-up looks better and goes on easier than it did with the regular moisturizer. My friends have noticed my **new** skin and say I look better than I have looked in a long time.*

D.S.B., Los Angeles

A. *It appears to really be fantastic. I am so impressed.*

J.M.D., Midland, Texas

A. *I had a few blackheads which have disappeared and skin appears clearer. Skin on throat is firmer. Skin is not dry anymore since using C-3 and C-2.*

R.B., New York